silver
LINING

Pam,
I am praying
fur you and with you
as you journey through
Cancerville. May God
keep you up beat
and your spirits
lifted.

*Cancer was the best
worst thing that ever
happened to me.*

God Bless,
Hannah McDonald
8/6/2020

silver LINING

*Cancer was the best
worst thing that ever
happened to me.*

Kommah McDowell

Printed in the United States of America

ISBN 978-1-0801-6026-6

This title is also available as an Amazon ebook.
Visit www.amazon.com/ebook.

Request for information should be addressed to:
QuestionsforKMI@att.net

All Scripture quotations are taken from the Holy Bible, New International
Version®, NIV®. Copyright © 1973, 1978, 1984 by Biblica, Inc.™ Used by
permission. All rights reserved worldwide.

Any internet addresses printed in this book are intended as a resource.
They do not endorse this book or Amazon in any way, nor does Amazon
vouch for the content on the referenced sites for the life of this book.

Cover design: *Doralynn Co*
                     Komodo Designs
                     dco@komodo-designs.com

DEDICATION

*This book is dedicated
to my village.*

We survived!

CONTENTS

FOREWORD

I met Kommah McDowell on April 18, 2018, at a City of Hope Spirit of Life Kick-off Breakfast. The event planning committee had decided to have a guest patient speaker that had been treated at City of Hope and that we could all be inspired by and learn from. I remember being introduced that morning to Kommah and remembering how her smile lit up the entire room. I had not known Kommah's story other than she was a breast cancer survivor and that City of Hope helped save her life. After a brief introduction, Kommah was invited to the stage.

As Kommah approached the podium to tell her story, what was abundantly clear was that she was not your ordinary life force. She was an extraordinary life force. Kommah was diagnosed with a rare form of breast cancer at a very young age and was given less than a 5% chance of living. And to make matters worse, they said if she did survive, she would never be able to have children. Fast forward 14 years to today, Kommah is completely healed.

Suffice it to say, you will find Kommah's story inspiring and a lesson for us all because as we face the darkest adversity in our lives, it is our perspective and love of family, friends and belief in our individual faith that gets us through to the other side where a bright light awaits. Kommah is a living, breathing example of that special light.

Evan Lamberg
President Universal Music Publishing
North America
President of The Board / City of Hope's Music, Film & Entertainment Division
Proud member of the Kommah McDowell Fan Club
May 19th, 2019.

Don't Quit!

This book was inspired by the poem, "Don't Quit", by an unknown author. While attending the University of California, Davis, this poem became the driving force of perseverance for me. I internalized this poem and I made it my own to get through college. Since then, it is this very poem that has carried me through many of the difficult times in my life when I wanted to just quit. Even through beating a rare form of breast cancer, to starting and dissolving a non-profit organization, and an attempted adoption, I did not quit. I thank God for giving me something to hold on to in those tough times. Perseverance is not easy, but it is often tested.

I have learned that in every situation there is always a silver lining if you just look for it. This book touches on several major events that have transpired in my life over the past fifteen years. Some of the events were so complex, I believe it is told best by including the thoughts and feelings of my husband, Charles McDowell Jr., my mom, Shirley Mordon, and my godmother, Tayja Mashack. With multiple vantage points, you will find how gracious God is, and there you will see the silver lining. I am stronger because of my journey and although I don't know what the future holds, I know what to look for to keep going.

For those who are not familiar with "Don't Quit", I have included it as a point of reference. I encourage you to meditate on this poem and allow it to resonate with you. For some, this may be just what you need. For others, this may be a simple reminder. But for all, the message is loud and clear, life is full of challenges that make us into the people we are today. Don't quit, it's just making you a better you.

Don't Quit

When things go wrong, as they sometimes will,
When the road you're trudging seems all uphill,
When the funds are low and the debts are high,
And you want to smile, but you have to sigh,
When care is pressing you down a bit,
Rest, if you must, but don't you quit.

Life is queer with its twists and turns,
As every one of us sometimes learns,
And many a failure turns about,
When he might have won had he stuck it out;
Don't give up though the pace seems slow –
You may succeed with another blow.

Often the goal is nearer than,
It seems to a faint and faltering man,
Often the struggler has given up,
When he might have captured the victor's cup,
And he learned too late when the night slipped down,
How close he was to the golden crown.

Success is failure turned inside out–
The silver tint of the clouds of doubt,
And you never can tell how close you are,
It may be near when it seems so far,
So stick to the fight when you're hardest hit–
It's when things seem worst that you must not quit.

You're too Young

"Anybody who has ever struggled to plant his feet onto the floor in the morning knows that life can be hard; it can be stressful; it can be overwhelming. But each of those negative, less than optimal feelings immediately takes a back seat to the inspirational power of hope."

Shawn L. Anderson, A Better Life

On July 15, 2005, in a small room, I laid on an exam table with a sheet up to my neck when the surgeon said, "I'm sorry, you have cancer." All of a sudden, everything became fuzzy and the only face I could see was my mom's. I said six words that still haunt her until this day, "Mom, how did I get cancer?" A tear fell from the corner of my eye. The room sat silent for what seemed like an eternity, until the surgeon's voice shattered the silence and reassured me that they were going to take care of me, despite the fact that they had misdiagnosed me for seven months. Now, understand, I felt the first aches and pains in December 2004. I was 28 years old. For seven months I had excruciating pain in my right breast, the color of the skin surrounding my right breast was bright red and resembled the texture of an orange peel. For seven months my right breast grew until it was twice the size of my left breast. For seven months, I was told by my female primary care physician that the changes I was experiencing were "normal" and that my hormones were the cause of it all. For seven months, I sat in my doctor's office every two weeks as each symptom invaded my body, hoping for answers. Yet, the only response I received was, it was my hormones because "I was too young to have cancer."

I recall asking my doctor, "Does your breast do what my breast is doing?"

"Does your nipple randomly invert?"

"Do you have discharge coming from your breast?" Which, by the way, was NOT mastitis?

"Was your breast so sensitive that no one could even brush up against your chest, let alone hug you?"

"Was there a lump the size of a plum under your arm, too?" A lump that made it unbearable to even rest my arm down by my side.

When asked those questions, my doctor said, "No."

I then asked, "So why is it normal for my breast to do all of these things, when yours doesn't? How is that normal?"

Thankfully, I had a Preferred Provider Organization (PPO) insurance plan and I was in control of my health. Fortunately, several years prior to this incident, I worked for a temp agency while I was completing my undergraduate degree. Who knew that that one placement would be a divine appointment that would ultimately change, if not, save my life years later? I was placed at USC Norris in a doctor's office that processed the paperwork for patients in need of bone marrow transplants. Sadly, I do not recall the name of the doctor I worked under, but what I do recall was some of the best advice I had ever received. The doctor told me at the end of my assignment, "When you get a "REAL JOB", make sure you get a PPO insurance policy, because if you ever get cancer you would be able to get the treatment you need without the red tape. It may cost you more upfront, but it will pay off in the end, if you ever need it." Wow!! *Who knew...* Fortunately, I never forgot his words and when given the first opportunity to obtain insurance, I did exactly what he said... *He was RIGHT!!*

So, with the confidence of having PPO insurance and out of pure frustration and great concern, I requested to have a mammogram. Sadly, I was told that a mammogram would not work for me because I was only 28 years old and my breast tissue was too dense due to my age. I was also told that as an African-American woman, inherently, it is common for my breast to have fibroid cyst and dense tissue, which makes it even more difficult to detect anything on a mammogram. Refusing to accept "NO" as an answer, I reminded my doctor that I had a PPO policy and I did not need her referral to do this. A few days later, I had my first mammogram, which was unbelievably painful due to the extreme sensitivity and swelling in my right breast.

A week later, I received the results from the mammogram. "The image is cloudy, but there were two lesions…" the report read. My doctor then went on to say,

"But it is not cancer because you are too young to have cancer."

As protocol would dictate, an ultrasound was ordered for more clarification. Unfortunately, that was inconclusive as well. The "ultrasound was consistent with a benign process, and a six-month follow-up ultrasound was recommended," per my medical records. My doctor explained to me that the ultrasound and mammograms were a bit hazy, but "nothing to be alarmed about because the unexplained growth was probably just a cyst they are not able to see on the films."

At this point, I did not know what to do. I began asking other women, including my mother, if what I was experiencing was normal. Of course, everyone insisted that something was wrong. With this affirmation, I was back in my doctor's office asking for her to help me, again. Sadly, she received me with great frustration. Sarcastically, she suggested a needle biopsy, which would be done in the exam room without any form of sedation. As scared as I was to hear the words NEEDLE and BIOPSY in the same sentence, I agreed, hoping to finally get some answers. Once I agreed, she excused herself from the room and then came back with a needle in hand. Startled by what seemed like a humongous needle, so many emotions flooded my mind and body. I was shocked, yet afraid, upset because I wasn't given any warning. My goodness, I wasn't able to prepare mentally for this moment. Not to mention, my older sister came to support me during this appointment and she is deathly afraid of needles. So, while trying to control myself, I am having to sooth my sister who was crying and screaming as if it were happening to her. Believe it or not, my sister helped me endure the biopsy. I was so worried she would hyperventilate during the process that I yelled at the doctor, "JUST DO IT! So she could stop crying." When the doctor stuck the needle into my breast and began to extract the fluid from what she thought was a cyst, nothing came out.

"Huh?" The doctor said with a puzzled look.

"Huh??" "What does that mean?" I said.

"Oh nothing." She shook her head and brushed it off.

I was so confused by her reaction and a little afraid because nothing came out of the cyst. Prior to the biopsy the doctor had shared that cyst are very common in the breast area, but they are just filled with clear fluid. There was nothing to worry about because most cysts do not require removal. But in my case, nothing came out… now what? Still, without confidence in my doctor, I eagerly awaited the results of the biopsy. A week later the results indicated no abnormalities. So again, despite the uncertainties of the mammograms, ultra sounds, and needle biopsy, I was repeatedly reassured that I only had a cyst because, according to my doctor, "I was too young to have cancer."

Finally, after months of doctors' visits and intense progression of whatever was "NOT" wrong with me, I asked for the cyst to be removed. My doctor was not in agreement with this request. She told me that she would schedule the surgical biopsy, BUT if it is JUST a cyst, she would no longer address this concern going forward. I graciously told her that I had a PPO policy and I had no problem finding another doctor after the biopsy. I felt trapped in so many ways. The last thing I wanted to do was start over with another doctor at this point.

In April 2005, I met with a surgeon to discuss his opinion on all the tests I had taken up until this point. He too reassured me that he believed I had a cyst and that it was against his better judgment to do a surgical biopsy.

"Something is wrong with my breast, so please remove what you think is "NOT" wrong with me, because I am in so much pain I can't sleep, work, or do anything. If it is a cyst, take it out so I can go back to being normal." I pleaded with him.

"Ok," he said, "but if this proves to be a waste of time, I will not go back in again."

"So be it!" I said. I was tired, frustrated, scared, and hurting in every way… *something had to happen because this wasn't normal.*

At this point in my life, I was now 29 years old. I had recently achieved my Master of Science in Leadership and Management from the University of La Verne. I had a "REAL JOB" in tax and financial services that I had been at for four years. I remember the moment I was offered insurance through my company, I was 25 years old. I was given a list of providers to pick from, which was foreign to me because the only health insurance I had known was under my mother's coverage. So, my first question to my human resources representative was, "which one is a PPO?"

She attempted to explain to me how insurance worked, and all of a sudden, she sounded like Charlie Brown's teacher… "wamp, wamp, wamp!" After listening patiently to her lengthy explanation, I repeated my question, "which one is a PPO?"

I explained that I was told by a cancer doctor to make sure I get a PPO. So again, I asked, "Which one is a PPO?"

With a chuckle, my rep simply said, "They all offer the PPO option; just pick which company you prefer."

Now that made more sense to me. Thankfully, I picked a policy that would grant me access to one of the most prestigious cancer research institutions in the world, City of Hope.

In addition to completing my education and launching the start of my career in the tax and financial services world, in March 2005, my boyfriend, Charles McDowell Jr., proposed to me. I was engaged to a wonderful man I had known for four years, he was my best friend. Subsequently, because of our strong friendship, once he proposed, we prayed about a date for our wedding and to everyone's surprise, it was schedule six months out. We figured since we were 29 years old and both of us wanted to be married by 30, why wait?

As excited as I was to be engaged, I was also terrified of my reality, what was wrong with me? My greatest fear was telling my fiancé that I had serious health issues with no answers. I feared it would be too much to deal with and he would change his mind. Prior to the surgical biopsy, all he knew was I had a lump under my arm and I was having some issues with my chest. I kept the information very high level, and on a need to know basis. I was embarrassed, ashamed, and afraid of losing him if I was not perfect or even normal, for that matter. So, when it was determined that I would need surgery, I felt it was time to bring him up to speed on everything. Understand, Charles and I were not intimate before marriage, so, he had not seen my chest, which made it easy to keep everything from him. By this time, it was June 2005 and we had been engaged for three months. After briefing him on my journey to identify the symptoms I was experiencing, I asked him to be there for the surgery with my mom. Without hesitation, he said, "of course." I was so grateful for his support, but I still feared the unknown. My surgery date was set for the next month.

Surprise

The world needs less heat and more light. It needs less of the heat of anger, revenge, retaliation, and more of the light of ideas, faith, courage, aspiration, joy, love and hope.

Wilfred Peterson

On July 13, 2005, I was prepped and headed into surgery. My surgeon reiterated his stance regarding my surgery and I told him, "just make sure I don't wake up dead." Minutes into the biopsy, the surgeon opened my breast and found something he wasn't prepared for. After extracting a few samples, he closed me up and headed for the waiting room to inform my mom and fiancé.

"It looks like cancer, but it is very bazaar" he said.

He had never seen anything like this. He couldn't confirm or deny that it was cancer; the biopsy was going to be sent out for testing. He then asked for my mom and Charles to make sure I was not alone when I came for the results. "Please don't tell her until we are certain it is cancer," he said to them. He then walked out of the waiting room and left them breathless.

Minutes later, I was wheeled into recovery. As I woke, I could see the distress on my mom and fiancés' faces. They told me, at the time, that they were stressed about the biopsy, but all went well and they would be okay. Little did I know, there was so much more to the story. After about an hour in recovery, the surgeon dropped in to inform me that he was sending the labs out and that I needed to follow-up with his office in two days.

Deep down in my soul, I knew something was wrong, but I was hopeful that it was JUST a cyst. For two long days, we waited for the results of the labs. I took notice of the fact that my mom and fiancé were unusually tired and withdrawn. I even commented a few times about how their aura had changed. I asked them if they were sleeping at night and if not, why? I had no idea that they were praying fervently and holding their breath for what would be the biggest fight of my life.

Then, on July 15, 2005, the whole world, my whole world, came to a screeching halt. We arrived early to my appointment. We were immediately ushered back to a room to wait on the surgeon. Then, we were moved to another room, and then another. After waiting for what seemed like an eternity, we were told the delay was due to the surgeon trying to clear his schedule for us. This was killer for my mom and fiancé, because it was at that point, they knew something was seriously wrong. Finally, the surgeon entered the room with his R.N. It was deafly silent for a few minutes when he asked me to lay on the table to examine my incision. As I laid there, I could sense his countenance was down, and five life changing, terrifying, unthinkable words fell out of his mouth… *"I'm sorry, you have cancer."*

Instantly, my mind shut down and like many others, all I heard the surgeon say was "you have cancer, but I have never seen this kind before" and again, I found myself with Charlie Brown's teacher, "wamp wamp wamp." The next thing I recall was the surgeon giving me surgery options. He claimed that he did me the favor of clearing his schedule so that he could operate on me immediately. His plan was to remove the cancer by way of a lumpectomy in hopes to spare my breast, but something had to be done right away.

I glared at him and asked him, "How can I trust you to remove a cancer you are not even familiar with, especially, when you did not believe anything was wrong with me to begin with?"

So many thoughts raced through my mind….

I knew something was wrong, I just knew it!! Breast Cancer… me… how? I was 29 years old, no family history…how did I get cancer?

Then a tear fell…. *"Get it together, Koko!"* I thought.

It was at that point I had to think… Then, the surgeon's R.N. saw my hesitation and gently said, you can always get a second opinion. Then, it hit me, City of Hope. I told the surgeon, "I want my records to be prepared so that I could get a second opinion at City of Hope." I did not want to proceed with surgery, especially since I had to fight so hard to get to this point, trust was broken.

I was told days later that the surgeon was startled by what he discovered because he had expected to just remove a cyst. The films and other test results did not indicate any cause for alarm, which was why he was so adamant about not doing the surgical biopsy. Fortunately, I was persistent and did not just wait another six months for another false ultrasound.

Within days of my diagnosis, I had my first appointment at City of Hope. Many have asked me how I knew to go to City of Hope immediately upon receiving my diagnosis. My mother worked in aerospace for 17 years and her office was *literally* around the corner from City of Hope. She used to come home and tell my sister and me about the place she would walk through on her lunch and breaks that was so serene. She talked about the Rose Garden, the Japanese Garden, the Garden of Statues, and the water fountain. She loved walking the campus with her co-workers, not knowing that someday she would be walking through the Rose Garden fervently praying for me. I credit my mother for initially introducing me to the ambiance of City of Hope through her descriptive words. However, it was during that same summer I learned about PPO insurance policies that my next assignment was at City of Hope in one of the bone marrow labs as an Administrative Assistant. It was then that I saw firsthand how doctors and researchers worked side by side. I was amazed at the level of engagement between those who were working to develop new medicine and those who were administering medicine. I was in awe of the intricate dance between colleagues at City of Hope as they cared for each person in need. My mom was right, there was something about City of Hope that made you feel hopeful by simply stepping foot on the campus. She was also accurate in her description of the Rose Garden, Japanese Garden, and main fountain... *serene*.

Hope

Hope is not easily defined, but impossible to embrace without faith. The more we search for meaning in what seems hopeless; we realize that our "hopelessness" is a state of mind, not a reality.

Carol Bright, Determined Means

On July 25, 2005, I entered the campus of City of Hope still in shock from my diagnosis from the other medical facility. My Nurse Practitioner, Cathy Cole, was the first person I met on my medical team. She was a breath of fresh air. Her gentle words and soft embrace showed me I was more than just another patient and she cared about me. She showed empathy, not sympathy for me and I appreciated that more than she knew. Next, I met Dr. Shen, my breast surgeon. She was the first doctor on my team that I met, and she was very empathic even to the point of making me feel like she came to work just to see about me. I felt comfortable entrusting my life to her and her team. This level of trust was quickly tested because after reviewing all my records and films, Dr. Shen met with my mom, fiancé, and me delivering another blow to my initial diagnosis. She explained that my symptoms and records appeared to indicate I had a rare form of breast cancer, Inflammatory Breast Cancer (IBC), but she was not absolutely certain. IBC is a type of breast cancer that starts in the skin of the breast and blocks the lymph vessels, then moves inward through the breast. It is fast moving and makes breast appear red and swollen, hence the name "inflammatory."

Fortunately, City of Hope had a doctor who was a specialist and she would consult with him and if possible, arrange an appointment for me ASAP. Dr. Shen was so amazing; she was able to get an appointment for me that very day. Unbelievably, an IBC Specialist was flying into City of Hope that same day to see his existing patients. He was one of a few specialists in the country that understood Inflammatory Breast Cancer in 2005. What a divine appointment!

A few hours later, we were introduced to the specialist, my future oncologist, Dr. George Somlo. Although we were warned that he may not be all warm and fuzzy, we quickly discovered he had a heart of gold. It was during this appointment where it was confirmed that I not only had breast cancer, but it was late stage Inflammatory Breast Cancer. I was told Inflammatory Breast Cancer is very aggressive. Not to mention, it was triple negative, therefore my hormones were not the cause for the cancer. According to statistics, in 2005, IBC was a disease with a 95% mortality rate. This aggressive cancer is typically found in younger women. Currently, if you were to Google Inflammatory Breast Cancer, you would see the statistics are still rather frightening, especially for African American women.

Fortunately, research continues and the rate of patients surviving beyond five years is growing. However, keep in mind, IBC survival is still very dismal when compared to the five-year survival rate of 98% for early-stage breast cancer. And, the survival rate for African-American women is even more daunting because we have the highest mortality rate for breast cancer, especially Inflammatory Breast Cancer. Not to mention, triple negative receptors, which present another challenge in treatment since triple negative tumors do not respond to standard hormonal therapy.

If that wasn't devastating enough, the possibility of having children was minimal. The chemotherapy I received typically sends women through early menopause. This meant my cycle would stop during chemo treatment. However, there was a 30 to 40 percent chance of my cycle returning. If it did, great, if not, not so great.

In looking back on this moment, I realize that Dr. Somlo was very empathic and he gave us the best-case scenario, which cracked the door to hope for us. In reviewing my medical records, it is clearly transcribed that I had a zero percent chance of having kids. Either way, having to deliver such horrific news to a young, engaged couple had to be heart wrenching for him too.

My heart sank, and I immediately looked at Charles. Silence overwhelmed the room. This was not our plan. We had talked about having four children and how we thought life would unfold for us. Little did we know that an atomic bomb was going to destroy everything we had hoped our future would be. Finally, I broke the silence and asked, "Is there time to freeze my eggs, just in case I beat this?"

Dr. Somlo said, "No, too much time has passed and you need to start treatment as soon as possible. Harvesting eggs is a lengthy process."

So, I had two choices, save my eggs or save my life. Well, when given those two options, Charles and I looked at each other and quickly agreed, "Let's move forward because we could always adopt." Ironically, we had already discussed adopting children at some point in our lives, so if that was the consolation prize, it was worth it to us. We both agreed, saving my life was the priority.

With that, Dr. Somlo provided us with additional details regarding what was to come. He arranged for surgeries, treatment, and scans. He reviewed more statistics related to the type of treatment regimen he had tailored for me, which we referred to as my chemo cocktail. At the close of our meeting, Charles, my mom, and I, were encouraged and we were ready to fight. As we stood up to leave, I told Dr. Somlo, "I know the statistics look bad, but if you just do your job well, God will do the rest." I honestly believed that God could make a way out of no way, so I wasn't so worried about odds and stats. We shook Dr. Somlo's hand and he escorted us out to the lobby.

Later that day, Charles shared with me that a year and a half prior to this moment, he had prayed to God asking if he would get married and if he and his wife would have children?

"The Lord promised that I would get married and that we would have children." He said with great confidence. He went on to say, "So because of that, I was not fazed by your diagnosis because I am trusting God, not man."

And so, the journey began…

Days after meeting Dr. Somlo and after so many conversations in my head, I recall the night I told Charles that I would understand if he decided not to marry me, and I gave him permission to leave with no guilt or shame. Honestly, who willingly signs up for a wife with a five percent chance of survival and, if I survived, not being able to have children because of the treatment process. I realized this was more than he signed up for when he proposed. But, Charles, being the amazing man that he is, looked me dead in my eyes and said,

"Are you crazy, I'm not going anywhere!"

He *chose* to go forward with marrying me, sick, bald and barren. Out of fear, love, and uncertainty, I cried myself to sleep that night.

The next morning, I was scheduled to have a quick surgery to implant a port-a-cath to help with chemotherapy (chemo) infusion. But, before we headed out for surgery, we received a call from a member of our church. My mom answered the phone, she stood silently with a blank stare, then she sat down. Charles and I paused; we could see the concern in her face.

"Oh no… ok. Thanks for calling." She said. She put the phone down and with tears in her eyes, she began to share the news she just received.

"One of your friends from church…" who was also a young adult, "was also diagnosed with Inflammatory Breast Cancer. She started chemo a few months ago…. Well, she passed last night."

"Oh no!" I thought. My mind began to wonder and I doubted the possibility of survival. I began to pray.

We all froze for a moment.

"I don't know who you two are referring to, but I do know that everyone is different and only God will determine if it is your time or not." Charles said.

"I know, you're right," I said. "We have to go now."

We were on our way to City of Hope and did not want to be late. The drive to City of Hope felt like forever. All we could think about was the news we had just received. It was then that we realized how narrow the survival window really was.

Surgery was quick, and it went well. My new port-a-cath was implanted just under my left shoulder. We headed home shortly after recovery. During the surgery, mom was given more information regarding my friend. She had a similar diagnosis of Triple Negative Inflammatory Breast Cancer with the same prognosis of a five percent survival beyond two years. This was devastating news and the timing was horrendous...

When news of this magnitude hits you, it is not uncommon to reach for anything that will help you stay afloat. I needed something to give me hope as I started my own journey of survival. For me, that was the book of Job in the Bible. I had read Job several times throughout my life, but NOW, I felt as if I was living it. I could personally relate to Job's suffering and I did not want to do it alone. I knew this journey would be a great testimony *and* I needed a support team to get me through it. So, I created an online study group that ventured into Job's world and looked at the similarities between what I was going through and what Job went through. This was my way of coping with my new reality. Interestingly enough, this was prior to technology being what it is today. We had email and group phone calls, but there were no social media platforms with immediate communication. So, with what was available to me, I organized an email-based study of the book of Job. It started with just family and a few friends. Then it multiplied rapidly to over 200 people as my journey was shared with others. It was amazing to see so many lives touched by what some would perceive as a horrible diagnosis. I was empowered by this and how so many shared their perspective of my journey, and why they choose to come along side me chapter-by-chapter, day-by-day, week-by-week. It was hard at times to accept the pain and emotional rollercoaster I was experiencing, but with so many supporting me, I was encouraged, determined, and sometimes pushed to press on.

Raw Emotions

"When you're in a dark place, you sometimes tend to think you've been buried.

Perhaps you've been planted.

BLOOM."

By Christine Caine

Below are my personal journal entries from 2005 after my diagnosis. I have been asked time and time again, how did I feel during my treatment journey? Fair warning, below are the intimate thoughts that flooded my mind when I was first diagnosed. I typed the selected entries verbatim to create a mental snapshot of where I was in the moment.

Job 1 - Entry   *8/1/2005*

Chapter 1 reminds me of what I am going through. There are so many obstacles in my life that are out of my control and my only recourse is to praise Jesus. I have had to deal with where I would get married, who will marry me, various roles in the church, and now cancer and individuals faking they are being supportive. One thing after the other and Lord, I felt you carrying me the whole way through. I am also grateful that I know you have picked me Lord, out of all of your other servants to be a vessel and spread the word and educate people. Thank you, Jesus. In this, I believe I have passed my first test as well. Satan will not get the victory because the victory is already won.

* * *

Job 2 – Entry   8/2/2005

My second test will be chemotherapy. I know many will want to come by just for comfort alone. I pray that I am as strong a person as Job and NEVER curse God. I know it will be trying, but in my weakness, He is strong. Also, I have an advantage over Job. I know I have to go through the treatment. I don't know how it will affect my body, but at least I know it is coming. In looking at Job speaking to his wife about cursing or not cursing God, I am reminded of how people expect me to be sad and down. People don't know how they would deal with cancer and automatically forget everything they were taught by Jesus and about Jesus. People act as if his healing power and deliverance is not for everything, only simple things. I literally believe that "by His stripes I am healed." But I also know that Jesus had to endure many painful, degrading, and terrible things for Him to get to the cross and die on our behalf. All I'm doing is fighting this cancer.

* * *

Job 3 - Entry   **8/3/2005**

*The day before my first chemo infusion.

    This chapter is quite interesting. I'm not sure how I will feel after the chemo treatment, but I pray it is not like Job. I don't want to curse myself or the day I was born. I believe that I was born for this moment and no matter how I choose to get here, I would see this very day one way or another. I am so very glad I chose you Lord, so that I know I've done my part in trying to live right and I am comforted by you throughout this entire experience. I am at peace, while others can't sleep. I am determined, while others are discouraged. I am hopeful, while others are afraid. You have allowed the storm to rage around me but not touch my spirit or my soul. I am a fighter because of the day I was born.

* * *

Job 3 cont...   **8/8/2005**

*4 days later...

    Thank you, Lord for day 4. Lord, knowing how Job felt in his misery, Lord I didn't ask why me. I never doubted you about myself and how strong I "really" was. I prayed for you to take the pain away and I told you and Cookie I didn't want to do this anymore. Father, I pray for continued endurance during this time. Although today is much better, I know chapter three will repeat itself several times before this is all over. I pray for the strength that you had to carry the cross all the way. I pray for the endurance and tolerance of pain. Lord, even writing hurts me now. I pray for guidance and proper use of my time on the good days. I pray for my care takers and their diligence and dedication. Give them the strength of Job's friends to just comfort when comfort is needed.

Thank you!

* * *

Job 4 - Entry   Date unknown

Eliphaz, like many I know, automatically assumed that Job did something wrong and made God mad at him. As I travel this journey, many people feel so sorry and sad for me. Therefore, they don't understand when I have good days and when my spirits are high. In Chapter 3, it was nice of Job's friends to lay in support of him without saying a word. That reminded me of the first Saturday after chemo when Cookie, mom, and Charles just sat with me in my room in the dark and they took turns all day. A blessing I had, which was different than Job, was my supportive friends and family trusted God and knew that this trial is a test of my faith. When they did speak, it was words of encouragement and motivation. They encouraged me when I became weak and wanted to throw in the towel. I am grateful to God for their support and clear understanding of the Lord's will.

* * *

Job 19:25 – I know that my redeemer lives, and that in the end he will stand on the earth.

Job 23:10 – But he knows the way that I take; when he has tested me, I will come forth as gold.

The Journey Begins

In fact, hope is best gained after defeat and failure, because then inner strength and toughness is produced.

Fritz Knapp, Vince Lombardi: Toughness

My first cycle of treatment was scary because of all the unknowns. We didn't know what to expect, what the room would look like. Would it be hot or cold? What did treatment look like, or feel like, for that matter? Was I going to feel the chemo going through my body? Would I be awake or asleep, would we talk or sit silently? So many questions, so many unknown answers. We did our due diligence by packing a bag filled with snacks, magazines, crossword puzzles, word searches, books to read, blankets, slippers, and something to drink. We were ready.

I was escorted to treatment by my Charles and my mom. After checking in to the clinic, we sat nervously in the waiting room for my name to be called. Minutes later it was time…

"Kommah," A nurse called from the side door.

I took a deep breath and looked at both Charles and mom.

"Yes, that is me!" I said, trying to be strong.

Greeted with a warm smile, the three of us were whisked back to the infusion room, which was my home away from home for the next four months during chemotherapy infusions. The infusion wing of City of Hope was much better than I had imagined. We had a private room with a TV. We had space to move around and eat. We had the option of opening and closing the door at our leisure. I laid down during most of the infusion because the first bag that was hung for me was Benadryl, just in case I was allergic to any of the medications I was receiving. I slept off and on as the nurse hung bag after bag.

The bags hung on shiny thin metal poles that came out the top of a small machine that beeped when the bags were empty. This machine sat on a thicker pole that flared out at the base with wheels underneath for easy movement. The bags resembled a jelly fish with long tubes that looked like tentacles which lead to the port-a-cath in my left chest. The fluids in the bag dripped to a slow cadence, one at a time, *drip... drip... drip...* A few of the bags were clear and they said saline, which was used to flush the tubes before and after my cocktail.

When the first clear bag was empty the nurse came into the room with a mask on wearing more protective gear as she hung a bag with red liquid and a large biohazard warning label on it. I did not know what was in this new bag initially, but after it was safely placed on the hook, she than began to explain that this was my chemo cocktail. After reconfirming I was the right patient for the bag she just hung, she attached the tentacles to my port. I sat and watched as the red drips patiently pushed out the saline and entered my body. I looked at the toxic warning, closed my eyes and prayed.

The side effects from the first chemo were so traumatic, my mind blocked out the details from the time I left the hospital to a week after treatment. Fortunately, Charles journaled a prayer for me two days after my treatment that sheds light on the events of the first week.

Courtesy of Charles' journal dated 8/6/2005.

Dear Lord,

This week Koko started chemotherapy on Thursday, 8/4, and the first day started off okay, but did not end all that well. Koko was tired, which was expected, and she was vomiting, which we think was caused by one of two things. Either, the food she ate, chicken and potatoes, or the medicine she took, since she chased it with liquid. So, her night was rough. Friday she was given a shot for her white blood cells to increase, which caused her body to ache. Her day was better than Thursday, which was a blessing. Lord, I have changed my prayer from what I want, to what you want. Lord, I don't like seeing her go through this pain and I ask for you to remove it. But, if that is not in your will, then I ask that you give her strength to climb.

My treatment regimen consisted of chemotherapy every 14 days and a white blood cell booster injection the day after each treatment. The cocktail for my treatment was very hard on my body and it caused me to be bedridden for 12 of the 14 days between treatments. It was as if I was paralyzed. Every two weeks I would have the strength to walk into chemo and four, six, or eight hours later, I was wheeled out to the car. During the 12 days between treatments, I would lie in bed with curtains drawn and blinds shut to minimize the risk of light piercing the darkness. Due to the chemo, I was also hypersensitive to light and sound. I had severe migraines and my body was riddled with pain to the point that my bed sheets hurt if they laid on me the wrong way.

Treatment was getting harder and harder. It seemed like the more chemo that dripped into me, the more pain and discomfort I experienced. About the third round of chemo, moving was not an option unless it was absolutely necessary. I thought I was surly going to die. I remember being in so much pain that I honestly did not believe I would see the next day. I prayed for my sins to be forgiven and I asked for my family and Charles to be ok without me, then I said the Lord's Prayer… with that, I drifted off to sleep forever, I thought. Surprisingly, I woke the next day. I was torn between being glad to see another day and wishing for the pain to just end. It was at this point I concluded that my body was at war with cancer and chemo. The goal and prayers were for the chemo to kill the cancer before it killed me. So many nights I thought the cancer was winning, but I kept waking up to see a new day. This journey literally taught me that tomorrow is not promised.

Hair Loss

"A positive statement propels hope toward a better future, it builds up your faith and that of others, and it promotes change."

Jan Dargatz, 52 Simple Ways To Give Your Spiritual Life A Lift

One of the greatest fears I had, once diagnosed with cancer, was the thought of losing my hair. I could not imagine myself bald. I tried to prepare myself mentally for the possibility of losing my hair, but at the same time praying to be in the small cluster of patients who beat the odds in hair loss. During the first week of treatment, I had many discussions around this topic and to help ease my mind, a nurse informed me that *if* my hair were to fall out, it would be about 14 days into my treatment. About day ten, after my first chemo treatment, subconsciously, I constantly ran my fingers through my hair. It was hanging between my shoulder blades, which was long for me, as I was growing it out from a short afro the year prior. My hair was very important to me because as a child my hair would not grow past my shoulders. So, having hair this long was a dream come true and I was very proud of it. Sadly, I could not imagine waking up one day with my beautiful hair resting on my pillow.

Being that I am not a gambler, I did not want to wait and see if my hair would fall out, I just knew it would... I figured I was not going to be the exception to the rule this time. Charles was very supportive during this process. He patiently weighed the pros and cons with me and said he would support either option. As sweet as he was, I recalled having candid conversations with him about how he loves long hair. Actually, it was my hair that caught his attention in church one day and lit the spark in his eye for me. He would often compliment me on how beautiful my hair was and he loved that it was getting longer. So, after much thought and discussion with my family, and knowing Charles loved my hair as much as I did, I knew it would be catastrophic if I just waited for it to fall out. Conversely, I decided to have Charles cut my hair back to a low afro to minimize the impact for both of us. Charles setup shop in my mom's garage; where I lived during our engagement.

As he began cutting row by row, tears fell from my eyes as the hair cascaded down around me. I was sad, so sad, and honestly, I thought he was too. However, we all knew it was best this way. But that didn't make it easy. When asked years later how or what Charles felt about this whole experience, he simply stated, "I supported you! Hair is just hair." He went on to share a dream he had prior to my diagnosis. He said in the dream, I had cut my hair off before the wedding. In retrospect, I recall him asking me out of the blue one day before I was diagnosed, "Are you planning on cutting your hair off?" My response was very nonchalant, "I don't plan on it." We believe, the dream prepared him for what was to come, which allowed him to be empathetic under the circumstances. That night, I cried. I was sad, but nowhere near as devastated as I believe I would have been.

Four days later, Charles came over to hang out with mom and me after work. As I sat on the recliner watching TV, my head began to itch. Like normal I scratched it, but this time when I pulled my hand back down it was full of hair. It was time... I couldn't breathe, I looked at my mom and Charles, slowly turned my hand towards them, it was full of hair and again the tears began to fall... With trembling hand, I rubbed my head and my hair slid off my head like a wig... *unbelievable*! I took a deep breath and said, "Wow!" But, of course, I had to have a stubborn patch of hair that refused to give in to the chemo. Smack dab in the center of my head, was an island of hair holding on for dear life. Unfortunately, it didn't last long, because Charles kindly shaved it off for me. This new look was different. So many thoughts raced through my mind.

How are people going to receive me?
What are they going to think?
I look like a boy with no hair.
Charles is going to hate this for sure!

Gratefully, the Lord had already prepared Charles for my bald head with his dream. He was very supportive and reassured me that I had a cute head with just a little hook. This was refreshing because I just knew he was going to hate it.

My mom on the other hand, I believe she took this very hard internally.

Knowing I was sick with no physical change made it a bit easier to bear. But now, seeing my hair on the floor, in my lap, slipping through my fingers, it was heart wrenching as a mother. She felt helpless. She recalled years later, she saw that in this moment, I was so strong and if anybody had to endure this, it was going to be me. However, this did not take away from the devastation she felt in her heart for me. She just prayed and prayed. As sad as she was, in the midst of praying one day, she had a particular moment when she felt a peace that surpassed all understanding and reassured her that I would be alright.

What a whirlwind of emotions one faces when your appearance is drastically altered. Now what??? Family and friends tried to be strong for me and encourage my new look by giving me pink skull caps, cute pink scarves, and hats. Little did they know, I hated the color pink! Nevertheless, before I knew it, I was drowning in Pepto Bismol pink EVERYTHING... journals, bags, pajamas, trinkets, blankets, shirts and so much more... Pink, Pink, Pink!! And my response to all the wonderfully pink gifts was, "Thank you for caring about me." I hated the color but loved the kind gestures. Quite honestly, today one would think my favorite color is still Pepto Bismol pink because after drowning in it for so many years, I realized it is a symbol of love, comfort, and support for me.

I made several attempts at wig shopping with friends and family to try and find a wig that would make me feel like "me" again. We sought long and hard for the perfect wig, but none of them came close to looking like my real hair. Early in my baldness, my sister said she would shave her head with me and we would be bald together. Understand, my sister is quite eccentric and she is not afraid of sparking a new trend with an edgy new look. In her mind, she had resolved that being bald was in and she was more than happy to rock it with me. I loved her so much for her enthusiasm and her desire to do this with me, but I told her not to do it. As amazing as she made the claim, *Bald is Beautiful*, I did not see it that way. To me, bald was sick and the last thing I wanted was for both of us to look sick. Sadly, I think deep down inside, I robbed her of an opportunity for her to show me how important I was to her in a tangible way as her little sister. But she respected my wishes and loved me through the journey in many other ways.

About two weeks into wearing wigs and growing more and more frustrated with them, my mom and I were walking though the mall and saw a young lady selling curling irons. For some odd reason, she was drawn to us and insisted on luring me in to test out her product on my wig hair. After declining the offer a few times, the poor girl never could have imagined what would happen next... I stopped, took off my hair and waved it at her.

"It's not real!" I said.

She gasped; tears filled her eyes, "I'm so sorry." She said in a shaky voice when she saw my bald head.

Not really knowing what type of reaction to expect, I laughed so hard at my baldness, but quickly realized I was the only one who found it funny. My mom hit my arm and glared at me. She then told me to never do that again. In the midst of my own internal battles about being bald, I did not consider the young lady and how she would respond to my foolish joke. In reflecting on her reaction, she was able to relate to my situation more than I knew. I realize now that it was easier to laugh at myself before someone could laugh at me. This was my way of saving face and protecting my pride, although, that was the last time I used that tactic.

Three weeks of hats, scarves, and wigs was enough for me to finally be tired of it all. I told everyone I didn't like wearing hats unless I am under an air conditioner vent and I really didn't like scarves on my head because they made me look and feel sick. I also hated wigs; they were too hot and itchy for me to wear all day long.

"I'm done hiding! It is time to just embrace my bald head." I thought.

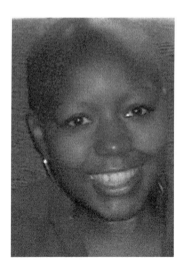

It was time for me to FINALLY look myself in the face and deal with my reality. As I carefully examined my scalp, I realized the shape of my head was cute, not too big and not too small. I had a cute hook on the back of my head, and having no hair made my eyes the focal point on my face. So, from that day forward, I wore cute earrings and eye makeup to enhance my beautifully bald head. It was freeing in so many ways, and I did not worry about what others thought- I was me! Charles and I joked that one day he would be as bald as me.

Embracing my baldness was freeing, but I still had to endure the staring eyes of strangers trying to process my appearance. Some asked why I choose my hair style. I would often explain it was because of chemo and that I was a cancer patient. These conversations often lead to people feeling sorry for me and or uncomfortable about the topic. Some feared I was contagious. Few were able to relate, but for the most part, people just stared from a distance, looking puzzled.

One day at about 8:00 a.m., I was home by myself and I heard a man's voice yelling outside of my window. I got out of bed and look to see what was going on, since I didn't have anything else to do. As I looked through my blinds, I could see a man yelling at a teenage girl from his car. He crept up slowly next to her as she appeared to be walking to school, jogging at times, to get away from him.

"Get in the car...I will take you wherever you need to go." He yelled through the passenger window.

The girl started panicking and tried to cross the busy street to get away from the man, but there was too much traffic. She was scared and was trying to run away, but the intersection was too busy for her to make it safely. After observing this situation for several minutes, I knew I had to do something to help this poor girl. So, before I knew it, I flew down the stairs in my pajamas and robe, through the garage, and down the driveway to the front of our gated community.

"LEAVE HER ALONE!!" I yelled at the top of my lungs.

Startled, the man and the girl looked directly at me. The girl realized this was her opportunity to escape, she quickly looked back at the street and saw there was a break in traffic, so she darted across the street without him noticing and hid. The man, however, was taken aback when he saw me.

He took a double take and yelled back, "Shut up you... you bald headed... B!#ch."

Suddenly, I realized I did not have a well thought out plan and that this man could now come for me. As fast as I could, I ran back in to the garage and closed it. I flew up the stairs to the middle landing and peaked though the blinds to see if the man was chasing me. Thankfully, he didn't bother me, but I could see him searching for the poor girl for a while, then he took off. She was gone. As scared as I was, I was glad I caused a diversion for the girl to escape.

A few hours after calming down and thinking about what just happened, I found myself doubled over in tears from laughing so hard at the man's face when he saw me. Being that I startled him, he wasn't expecting to see a bald lady in a robe with no shoes yelling at him through a gate. His hesitation, "you… you… bald B" became hysterically funny to me. That was classic!

On a side note, chemo not only affected my appearance. It took a toll on my taste buds too. Unfortunately, seasonings and spices exacerbate the desire to vomit, so it is highly recommended to eat bland foods during treatment. So, my two foods of choice were rice with milk, cinnamon, and sugar heated up in the microwave and flash-cooked oatmeal made with water. My poor caregivers had the daunting task of making the perfect bowl of oatmeal for me at my most miserable times during treatment. I recall Charles attempting to make oatmeal the way I like it one morning. After the fifth failed attempt, we couldn't take it anymore, so I got up and went downstairs and taught him how to make oatmeal my way. He was shocked to see the process was much quicker than he expected… Just put the oatmeal in hot water and let it set for a few minutes… then add sugar, DONE! He was disgusted, relieved and humored by this new discovery.

A few days after Charles' oatmeal lesson, my cousin-in-law came to care for me during the day while everyone else was at work. She was very attentive and did well handling me with care; however, she too was tested with making oatmeal for me. After her second failed attempt, she was wise enough to call Charles in her frustration. He told her, "Girl, just put the oatmeal in hot water, add sugar, and give it to her." Ten minutes later, she called him back laughing because she couldn't believe I ate it. It is funny how chemo heightens your five senses. Food textures were much more important than ever before, which was the case with the texture of the oatmeal.

My Village

There is always hope for a new day, hope that the darkness won't always seem impenetrable. There is always hope because our Redeemer lives.

Marcia Laycock, Celebrate This Day

I have always been told "it takes a village to raise your children" I can honestly say; my mom believed this expression wholeheartedly and she made sure my sister and I were surrounded by a village she could count on. As a child, my family lived at church, St. Stephen Missionary Baptist Church in La Puente, CA., five if not six days a week. We loved it! Our social fabric was stitched together at church. With choir, mission projects, bible study, birthday parties, friends, and "play" extended family members, this was our village since I was five years old.

I recall the Sunday after being diagnosed going down to the front of the church and asking for everyone to pray for me as I openly shared my diagnosis. As one who strongly believes in prayer, I figured this was a pretty good time to solicit as much prayer as possible and to not feel shame or embarrassment by my circumstances. Sadly, I learned through my journey, many diagnosed with cancer feel as if they did something to deserve their diagnosis. I knew I was not at fault in any way nor was I too proud to recognize when I needed support.

Fortunately, I had several play moms, family and friends in my village, physically and spiritually. I am forever grateful for Momma Bruner, Momma Rhonda, Sister Dawkins, Sister Starr, Sister Lawrence, Aunt Jackie, Shani, Momma Janice, Aunt June, co-workers, prayer warriors, and so many more I apologize for missing.

My family and I were overwhelmed with support, but one particular lady rode the waves with my mom and Charles moment by moment, my godmother Tayja Mashack. This lady was a pillar for my family. She was one of my main escorts for treatment and my advocate when my Charles or my mom were not available. She was present every step of the way, just as if I were her very own.

Years after this experience, I became curious about my godmother's perspective regarding this time in my life, our lives. In response, she shared the following:

I remember the day well when you called me and told me you had cancer. In that moment, I felt helpless! We had been having so many conversations about life and love. Never thought we'd have to share the experience of you going through cancer treatment. One phone call changed my life! It showed me how vulnerable all of us are to this disease called cancer. My thoughts went in many directions and I had to focus in on what I could do to help you through this faith building exercise!!

When I went with you to treatment, I will never forget how challenged I felt with them giving you a medicine that had an X and poison on the cover. It took me by surprise the first time I saw it. I really had to talk to myself and say this is a necessary medicine so my baby can get well. As your godmother, I really had a problem with why we (your family) would let someone give you poison to get well.

I remember one of the times I was at the house

and you had just had an IV treatment. Charles and your mom were trying to cover the window with dark material because your eyes were sensitive to the light. My heart broke for a minute; it took me back to allowing the doctor to put poison in your body. I cried all the way home. Wishing I had a way to take this challenge away from you. If I was feeling this way, I'm sure your mom and your fiancé at the time, had their moments too.

I remember the conversation we had when Anne Sevier died with the same type of cancer. When you first found out, your mind started wondering about your own mortality. At that point, we, your village, had to ask you to be selfish for a moment and concentrate on you! It didn't mean we didn't want the best for Anne, I just felt if you focused in on her, it would be difficult to see God work a miracle in your life, and just focus in on yourself. I was constantly in contact with Sarah Adams at that time...praying for Anne and making sure if there was anything I could do I would.

However, I knew that God set-up our relationship long before you were diagnosed so that during this time you would feel my heart! Know how much I loved you and that I would do anything to make sure you survived cancer. I remember asking your mom if she was ok with me being your godmother. I felt it was such an honor to be chosen for such an intimate *relationship with you. When she said yes, I was grateful and pleased to be your godmother! I love you so much!*

As expected, cancer had taken a toll on my body, mind, and definitely tested my spirit, but I wasn't the only one going through it. My village struggled along side of me through my entire journey, especially my Charles. My Charles was my rock! He drove me to and from my appointments when available, he sat through the surgeries with my mom, time after time. He organized a caregiver schedule for tons of people to keep me company at home, during infusion, and recovering from surgeries. He changed my drains when needed, was a short order chef for my bland palette, washed my clothes, sanitized my room and bathroom, shopped for any particular necessity, changed bandages, logged all medications, fevers, side effects, treatment, and meals, paid all the bills, mine and his, kept me company when I was awake after work, and maintained the high demands of his daily job. He was my Superman!

I Did, So I Do

Sometimes the world around us seems empty, and we may feel entirely alone, but now and then - Suddenly! - when we least expect it - when we've almost given up hope - when we're tired or bored or fearful or disgruntled - God breaks through and the angels start to sing.

Ray Pritchard, Joy to the World!

Chemo was very challenging for me, my family, and my support team. But, to add to our day-to-day challenges, I was still engaged and had a wedding to plan that was set for October 29, 2005. I remember in September, one month into treatments, telling Dr. Somlo that I was getting married, bald and all, on October 29, so I needed him to adjust my treatment schedule to accommodate for the wedding and honeymoon. After he realized I was serious, he so graciously adjusted my schedule so that I had three weeks between my infusions, as oppose to my standard two weeks, which allowed me to take a three-day honeymoon before heading back into treatment. I am so grateful I wasn't just another patient or number, but a member of my medical team at City of Hope. My input was considered and made a difference, which made my journey that much easier.

Many concerned family and friends tried to convince Charles and me to wait until after my treatment was done to get married. But, after the blessing from my medical team and with few restrictions, we kept the date. However, I was not allowed to touch guests and I had special cooking requirements for my food at the reception. In addition, I had to figure out how I was going to walk the day of the wedding, especially since our venue had six flights of stairs that led down to where the wedding ceremony was taking place.

Prior to my diagnosis, Charles and I had secured Coco Palm's, a Cuban restaurant that cascaded down the east side of a hill overlooking the San Gabriel Valley, for our wedding ceremony and reception. Six marble stairways gracefully flowed into the wedding ceremony platform where the trees formed the perfect arch. Coco Palm's was a dream location for a wedding with unobstructed breathtaking views. Little did we know, six months later, walking would be my greatest challenge on our special day.

Days before our wedding, I found myself still struggling to walk after treatment. At our wedding rehearsal, on October 28th, it rained. We practiced me being carried down the six flights of marble stairs to the base of the last flight. Then, from that point I would be wheeled into the ceremony. But this was not the vision I had for my wedding day. I was not okay with being carried into my wedding.

I told everyone, "I WILL walk tomorrow, if it is the last thing I do. I WILL NOT be carried into my wedding like I am sick…I can't do that."

That night, Charles and I prayed for two miracles, (1) I would walk and (2) for the rain to stop just long enough for us to get through the ceremony. For the past week, it was expected to rain like cats and dogs. We had grappled with having the patio area for our wedding ceremony enclosed with a canopy. Literally, three days before the wedding as it was pouring down outside, we sat in the caterer's office and agreed to take our chances. As usual, everyone thought we were crazy for not utilizing the backup plan. Our rationale was, God *could* part the clouds for us on our special day, so we prayed. The next morning, our wedding day, I recall waking up to the weather report on the local news.

"I'm not sure what happened. It was supposed to rain all weekend but the sun is out, and the rain is gone." The weather man said.

I was so excited when I heard this, I jumped out of the bed and ran to the window and threw the blinds open. The phone rang, it was Charles.

"Did you look outside yet?" He asked.

I laughed and told him, "I am standing in front of the window as we speak!"

We were so amazed at how beautiful the morning was. I was so excited, I ran and jumped back in the bed thanking God for parting the clouds on our special day. Then, it hit me… Wait, I walked… I WALKED!! I couldn't believe it, I was walking and running. WHAT!!! I called Charles back and screamed with joy, "I'M WALKING, I'M WALKING!!" Tears filled my eyes, I couldn't believe it.

A friend was staying with me in a hotel room that night and she sat frozen when she first saw me move. She was in shock and she didn't want to startle me. Then she pleaded for me to stop walking and rest to save my energy. It was a miracle!

As the wedding party began to arrive, they could not believe I was walking. Everyone, including me, was nervous because we did not know how long my strength would last. So, we took precautions by having me sit as often as possible, we even sat during the ceremony and through pictures. But, when it was time for me to enter the ceremony, I WALKED, slowly, down all six flights of stairs with the assistance of my cousin and brother-in-law. I DID IT!!

Charles and I had planned a choreographed dance to Alicia Key's *If I Ain't Got You* prior to my diagnosis, but we were not able to practice once my treatments began. A few days before the wedding, we agreed, if I were up for it, we would do what we could remember of the dance during our reception. For us, the dance was a lyrical depiction of our relationship. The lyrics to the song really expressed how we felt about each other, especially under the circumstances. I was feeling good and did well through the ceremony and pictures. I kept asking myself, "are you okay to dance?" So, not only did I walk into the ceremony, but we were able to dance our dance for our family and friends with the last bit of energy I had. As tired as I was, I felt AMAZING!!

As the lyrics flowed, so did we...

Some people live for the fortune

Some people live just for the fame

Some people live for the power, yeah

Some people live just to play the game

Some people think that the physical things define what's within

And I've been there before, and that life's a bore

So full of the superficial

Some people want it all

But I don't want nothing at all

If it ain't you baby

If I ain't got you baby

Some people what diamond rings

Some just want everything

But everything means nothing

If I ain't got you, yeah

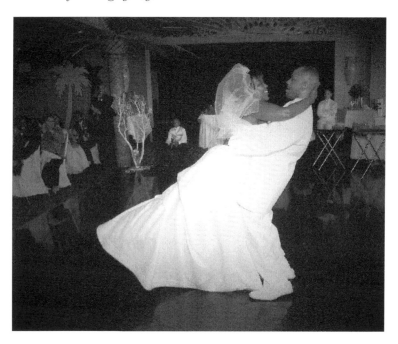

Some people search for a fountain

That promises forever young

Some people need three dozen roses

And that's the only way to prove you love them

Hand me the world on a silver platter

And what good would it be

With no one to share, with no one who truly cares for me

…So nothing in this whole wide world don't mean a thing

If I ain't got you with me baby

By Alicia Keys

Charles choose to support me through this journey, not many men would have done what he did. As a matter of fact, we later learned that the divorce rate is six times greater for women with cancer. Understanding there are many dynamics that play into divorce, battling a terminal disease is very taxing on a relationship. Nevertheless, less than a week after our wedding, I was headed back in for treatment. Escorted by my *new husband*, we entered the infusion area and to our surprise, we received a standing ovation from the nurses and techs. Several people shook Charles' hand and told him that he was a "good man" to marry me under these circumstances. They shared how they often have to console patients who have been left by their significant other because taking care of them was too much to bear. We were told that it was rare that a patient would actually get married during treatment with a terminal diagnosis. We were different!

Not only were we different, but the type of cancer I had was different. For Inflammatory Breast Cancer, surgery is done post chemotherapy. One of the many unique characteristics of Inflammatory Breast Cancer is the fact that this fast-moving cancer is also in the skin of the breast and within the breast. Therefore, chemo is used to slow down the rapidly growing cancer cells, with the hopes of stopping them completely prior to surgery. In my case, I had a radical right mastectomy with lymph node dissection. Or in other words, my right breast and lymph nodes were removed. My breast surgeon, Dr. Shen, was phenomenal. She was able to remove all the necessary breast tissue and stitched me back together very respectfully. As grateful as I am for her skilled hands, I was still left with grappling with only having one breast at 29 years old.

After my first mastectomy, I remember being afraid to look at my chest in the mirror. I stood in the bathroom with my face down when my husband walked in and encouraged me to look up. He reminded me, my scars are my signs of survival and to not be ashamed of them. I face daily challenges with body-image because of the visual and mental scars post treatment.

Perseverance

"I hope if you have doubts about yourself, you'll be able to re-evaluate your old beliefs and rediscover the amazing person you've always been."

Sandra V. Abell, Feeling Good About You

After recovering from surgery, I went back to work while undergoing radiation therapy. Although this was not as hard on my body as chemo, the radiation burned my skin until it turned charcoal black. I was often fatigued from the radiation, but I was glad to return to some sense of normality. My hair started to grow back and I was beginning to look like my old self again. I was excited to be on the other side of chemo. To celebrate, my family and I signed up for a Revlon 5k Walk in Los Angeles, CA. We were so excited; we invited others to join us as a celebration of life. To our surprise, our team grew to include over 100 people. Our team name was, Praying For A Cure! And we even had a huge banner made to lead the way.

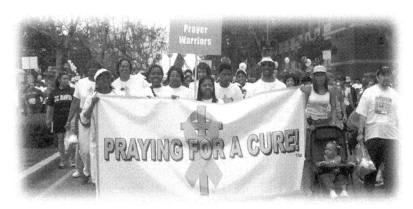

We found ourselves energized by the 1000's of people participating in the walk overall. However, I was concerned about my ability to make it to the finish line. Just before the walk was underway, I began to doubt myself. Knowing that I was still recuperating from treatment and surgery, in addition to actively undergoing intensive radiation therapy, I worried that this would be too large of an endeavor.

"I may not be able to make it through the full 3.1-mile walk. But, since the course goes through the streets near Exposition Park, you could leave me on a bench and come back and pick me up in the car after the walk." I told Charles and my mom.

I'm not sure if they knew how serious I was, because neither one of them responded to my comment. It was like they both just ignored me.

"POP"

"POP"

"BANG!"

"And they're OFF!" Exclaimed the announcer.

"Let's do this!" Charles encouraged.

I just looked at him and said… "Ok, let's go!"

About halfway through the walk my body was exhausted. My legs began to hurt, my breathing was inconsistent, and mentally I was looking for a bench to wait on.

"I'm sorry, I don't think I can make it. Just find a bench and I will wait here. It's almost over so you shouldn't be too long." I said.

As soon as I spit out the last word, I heard heavy breathing coming from behind me. Then I heard *click click* pause, *click click* pause, *click click* pause.

"What is that?" I thought.

A few minutes later, an elderly gentleman with a frail frame began to pass me. He had two crutches and one leg. He was breathing hard, but he seemed to be galloping to a cadence, *click click* pause, *click click* pause. He was determined and focused. He didn't even look up, he just kept to his cadence, *click click* pause, *click click* pause. As he passed our group, which was walking at my pace, everyone's eyes followed him, *click click* pause, *click click* pause, until he was out of sight. Then, they looked at me.

"Thank you, Lord for giving me a reality check. If that man is able to endure the walk with one leg and crutches, how dare I complain about my legs hurting. I will not complain another time. We are almost there." I declared.

It took everything in me to muster up enough strength to make it to the finish line, but I did it! For weeks after the walk all I could hear in my head was *click click* pause, *click click* pause. I became inspired by that man who did not allow his circumstance to dictate his ability. He did not succumb to his disability; he just found another way to succeed. Now that was the epitome of living to me. With God's strength, that is who I needed to be. Despite the statistics, limitations, circumstances, and excuses, I needed to stay focused and find a way to succeed.

Body Image

"Even your past pain can be a blessing to someone. Hopelifters are willing to reach back and pass hope on."

Kathe Wunnenberg, Hopelifter

After nine long months, I was completely done with treatments. Charles and I were finally going to get our chance to have a "normal" life as newlyweds with one caveat. We were reminded that I would not be able to have children, but just as a precaution, we were told to use protection until I was at least two years post treatment. We agreed! We knew statistically, my survival rate was five percent within the first two years of diagnosis. Also, we were told, if the type of cancer I had were to return, it would come back with a vengeance. Therefore, my medical team wanted to be able to treat me without worrying about a baby too. This was a hard pill to swallow but was understandable.

So, with this information and my tired, fatigued, and scarred body, I realized I was not able to do the things I used to do. What used to be "normal" for me, in some cases, was not even possible anymore. I struggled trying to do things and learned that I needed to establish a "new normal" for myself. I had to accept the limitations that came with my survival. Initially, I found myself frustrated by my limitations until I realized how selfish and childish, I was being. Tomorrow isn't promised to anyone and the fact that I was still alive was worth the limitations. I learned to live within my limits and sometimes, I pushed them.

My "new normal" consists of limited movement from all the scar tissue under my arm and tightening of skin from my mastectomy. Fatigue when I pushed myself too hard for too long. Limited physical endurance, a lower immune system, and a lower sex drive. I am the *one* in 1,000,000 who gets most of the side effects for most medicines. So now when I get sick, I must ask about all side effects before accepting medication. If the side effects listed are too severe, I have to ask for an alternative medicine. My memory glitches often due to Chemo Brain, *which is a real thing,* so I have had to learn to take notes and make lists. As for intimacy with my husband, well, that was another challenge.

With all of the scars, neuropathy, and only having one breast, I had no self-confidence. I became ashamed of my body, probably to the point of a mild depression. Intimacy became a major concern with my husband and me. Sadly, I completely lost the desire for any form of intimacy. Touch represented pain in my mind, even gentle touch. After being in some form of pain for so long, the desire to be touched was gone. Fast forwarding a few years, you will learn that this issue resurfaced several times throughout my journey, and will probably continue throughout my life.

Over time, I permanently lost complete feeling in my breast, upper part of my arms, sides, and lower abdomen. I was and still am physically deformed from all of the surgeries I have endured. Thus, our intimate times together became more of a contractual obligation. I did what I was supposed to do to satisfy my husband, no more, no less. The experience was not enjoyable at all, actually, it was rather painful in most cases. If you had asked me, I thought my insides had just dried up all together and were incapable of being aroused. We tried all sorts of tricks and tips, but nothing seemed to work. Intimacy was frustrating!

Not surprising at all, Charles was equally frustrated with our time together. He felt lost, like a virgin, rediscovering things in which he had just learned about me and my body prior to my major surgeries. He had no clue as to what to do with me. Where to touch, not touch. What to say or not say in fear of hurting my feelings. He introduced artificial lubrications, in hope to make the experience more pleasurable, but to no avail. We learned about lymphedema massages to reduce the swelling in my arms and back. He was trained on how to incorporate the massage into our time together, in hopes that it would not only relieve pain in those areas for me, but prayerfully, it would cause some type of arousal. Sadly, it was more relief than anything. Charles was very aware of the fact that I had no sex drive at all. He knew I was just doing my duties as a faithful wife, but never did I initiate it, nor did I care for it to last any longer than it had to.

At first, I thought it was just me, and I started to become withdrawn from

Charles, which was scary. He was my best friend and the ONLY man I would ever want to be with. We knew statistically, so many marriages fail over sex and money. We vowed to not fall into those statistics, but before we realized it, we were standing in quicksand. Knowing that something had to change, I started talking to people I trusted about my issues and concerns with intimacy. After discussing my concerns with my medical team, I was relieved to learn that this was a typical side effect for women who had experienced similar treatments and surgeries. My godmother, Tayja Mashack, was very helpful in grounding me with this issue. Without apology and very sincerely, she gave me what I believe was sound advice.

"As a wife, it is your job to make sure the needs of your husband are met." Without skipping a beat, she went on to say, "I have always felt that you should always come up with a way to provide intimacy with your spouse in whatever way is necessary. The word says the marriage bed is undefiled. Which means, you are to do what needs to be done for your spouse to feel satisfied. Intimacy doesn't always mean the complete sexual act. It means what will work for the two of you in the privacy of your relationship. Men have needs that need to be met and as his wife, it is your responsibility to meet them. No excuses. He is a man, if you don't fulfill his needs, someone else will try to do it for you." Her voice softened a bit, "I know you are not feeling well all the time, but that doesn't change the fact that you have a husband and he has needs too. On your good days, you have to make the best of it."

I was not shocked by my godmother's advice; she speaks from a place of wisdom and she is not into dancing around issues. She hits them head on EVERY time. She doesn't fall for excuses and she has no problem calling me on the carpet when it is necessary. She would always tell me, "I am too old to be playing games. I don't have time for it." I loved this about her. She is a no-nonsense woman with grace. What others may not have known, but she saw very clear, was I used my sickness as an excuse because I lacked the drive for intimacy. I thought it was justifiable if I didn't feel like being touched, considering I associated touch with pain. Sadly, my husband was taking the brunt of many surgeries that left me with neuropathy, pain and discomfort or severed nerves that wreaked havoc on my body. My nerves in my chest constantly sent misfire signals to random parts of my body. This in turn resulted in having many hours of trying to scratch phantom itches, which resulted in more pain and zero satisfaction. Charles could not compete with my internal struggles.

After processing my godmother's advice and praying for the intimacy to return, Charles and I had to have a hard conversation about how uncomfortable I was in our coming together. We discussed that my sense of touch was drastically different than it was when we first got married. You see, I was only halfway through treatment when we married. I had both breast and the swelling and pain was under control. Short of poison running through my body and being bald, I was normal. I did not have side effects that affected my sex drive because I was still in treatment. So, on my good days, we had some *GOOD NIGHTS*... It is surprising how one could be so spoiled after a short period of time. Actually, I am sure Charles would beg to differ. He would probably say the addiction started the very first time on our wedding night.

Thankfully, Charles is very intuitive and he suggested that we start over. He too had been seeking godly council on our lack of intimacy. He told me that the best advice he had received was for us to take time to learn new erotic zones on my body with touch. I remember the evening we sat on the bed, fully clothed and engaged in one of our hard talks. Charles then explained our new plan of action and how we would start over. Starting over meant, he literally explored my body to determine my reaction to his touch. By doing this, we realized the severity of scars and the scar tissue left behind. We had to modify our way with each other to ensure our time together was pleasurable for both me and him. This was quite difficult because I had to allow myself to be vulnerable to him and to trust that he would handle me with care. We took our time through the process, we laughed at times, I cried a little, but overall, we were in a better place. In retrospect, this was another critical moment in our relationship that we were able to maneuver through together. Despite shame, guilt, and embarrassment, it was worth it. So, this is me, my new normal.

My Legacy

"I hope you find grace in this world, that you recognize your worth, and that you can shine."

Tsang Lindsay, Live Free: Re-Write Your Story

"If we expect change, we must act on our hope every day until we have accomplished what we wanted."

Christopher Goodman, The Best Life Lessons, Inspirations and Quotes

As grateful as I was for my job and the wonderful insurance I had, I started to long for something more from life. I knew that the odds of me seeing the next few years were minimal, so I had a desire to create a legacy support. I thought about the patients I encountered in the waiting rooms and infusion rooms who were unaccompanied by anyone. There were a few patients who would get dropped off, sit or lay for hours during chemo infusion, and then get wheeled out to a car for a ride home. No one interacted with these patients, aside from the treatment staff and oncologist. They had no family or friends keeping them company. Another patient I observed was a single mother with a young child. I overheard her speaking with someone about not having enough money to continue treatment because she needed to be able to provide for her child too. She pleaded her case of not being able to pay for transportation to get to treatment because she needed the money to keep a roof over her child's head.

I was devastated!! In one situation, some patients find themselves walking through one of the most terrifying journeys of their life alone. Not feeling loved or supported when you are most vulnerable and have the greatest need is unimaginable. Then, to watch this poor lady have to choose to die because she could not afford to live, is deplorable! I felt horrible because I had such a huge support team surrounding me. I had caregivers with me around the clock. During my six- and eight-hour infusions, I would have two to three people tag teaming to watch me sleep through infusions so that when I woke up, I was not alone. I had co-workers providing meals for my family on infusion days so that my family did not have to worry about cooking on those days. I had friends and church family buying me comfortable clothing to help with the hypersensitivity I was experiencing from the side effects. I had all the wigs, scarves, hats, and socks I could ever desire. I knew I was loved, supported and cared about. But that was not the case for others and that broke my heart.

I have always been one to fight for the underdog. Cancer patients who were in need of resources and support were worth fighting for. So, after significant research and planning, Charles and I decided to start a foundation in my name to help cancer patients. Our goal was to leave a legacy that poured love into the lives of cancer patients who had a need. The organization was going to focus on the day-to-day needs of families in the trenches of treatment. It would include, food, transportation assistance to and from treatment, utility bills, and prescriptions. It would also include assistance with rent or mortgages. This organization would represent the support team I had during my treatment journey so that others would know they were loved and supported too. We named it, Kommah Seray Inflammatory Breast Cancer Foundation (KSIBCF).

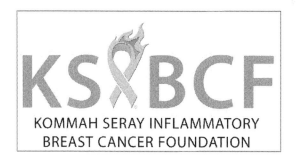

I developed a plan to launch KSIBCF to the cancer community. Grateful to have a Bachelor of Arts in English from the University of California, Davis and Master of Science in Leadership and Management from the University of La Verne, I was able to construct the organization structure of the nonprofit and ensured that it was aligned with the best practices of similar successful nonprofit organizations. In the summer of 2006, I wrote the business plan for KSIBCF and in October 2006, we received official documentation that KSIBCF was cleared for business.

Our founding board consisted of Terri Whiting, PA as Chair of the Board, Eleanor Monroe, CT, MPA as Co-Chair of the Board, Angela Urrutia, Founding Partner of SIU, LLC as Secretary of the Board, Tayja Mashack, Owner of Mashack & Pauley, INC as Treasurer of the Board, and Dr. Susan Nyanzi, DrPH, CHES, Chronic Disease and Wellness Specialist, Charles McDowell Jr, and Vanci Fuller, Esq. as Members of the Board. I served as the Founder and Executive Director of KSIBCF. The foundation served two purposes; to raises awareness of Inflammatory Breast Cancer and to offer support to cancer patients in treatment. We figured we had two good years to set the groundwork for this organization while I was healthy enough to help build the legacy. We knew we were working against an unofficial count down of a looming statistic within a two-year survival rate.

The first six months, KSIBCF started like most home-based, grassroots organization. As much as I loved working from home, it was becoming more and more challenging separating home life from work life. So, the Board, Charles, and I began praying for an affordable office space. After a few weeks, Vanci Fuller arranged for KSIBCF to rent out a small office within her law firm's office space. It was located in a high-rise in Covina, CA and it was unbelievable in so many ways.

The layout and the furnishing dictated professionalism and confidence. Guests were greeted with a quaint waiting area upon entry. It was furnished with an inviting sofa, chair and a table with magazines to peruse through once they had check in with the receptionist. With cherry wood furnishings throughout and high back office chairs, the first room was a large formal conference room with a huge polished oval table, then three smaller offices with glass walls followed in a row. The corner office over looked the main street and the shopping center across the way. The remaining two office spaces shot to the right of the corner office, both equal in size. The space also included a mini-kitchen and two storage rooms. Our two office spaces were nestled between the conference room and the corner office. I was amazed at how God set KSIBCF up in such a distinguished and professional space for our first official office. Subsequently, as our space grew, so did the needs of the foundation. Within a few months of settling in, I gained two additional volunteers, Olivia Williams and Helen Lawrence, who were amazing friends from church. They helped get the foundation rooted in the community.

As we delved further into KSIBCF, we discovered the underbelly of the cancer community that only seemed to exist for those who are deeply impacted by cancer. As KSIBCF was coming to fruition, I became more aware of the various dimensions of what I call, Cancerville. My journey to Cancerville began as a patient and progressed to becoming a professional Patient Advocate. As you may recall, upon the discovery of my initial diagnosis, I experienced discrimination by my primary care physician and the surgeon who performed the first biopsy. They both disregarded the possibility of me having breast cancer because of my age. My primary care physician repeated her stance of, "you are too young to have cancer," every time I showed up in her office over the course of seven months.

As a young patient, I thank God that I trusted my body and not my doctor. I learned early on in my journey, it was not uncommon for young adults to experience this type of discrimination with medical concerns. This realization was like the commercial when the M&M's and Santa Clause saw each other for the first time, and they both said, "He really does exist" and then faint. Ageism exists, and it was more common than I could have ever imagined. I had to do something, say something, change something.

After working tirelessly for five years, KSIBCF was finally in a position to secure our own office space. With growing programs and events, we began to overtake the law office. Financially, we were ready for the next step. So, in 2012, KSIBCF had a store front office that was more client friendly. The layout included an open work space where we placed two desks, two private offices, an open conference room, a restroom, and a kitchenette. Our new space also lead to increased exposure. It granted easier access for clients and supporters. It was a comfortable environment for clients in vulnerable

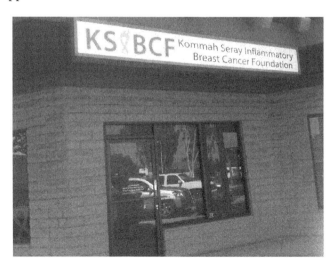

situations and had a playroom for clients with children that evolved over time into a Free Clothing Boutique.

As a survivor of Inflammatory Breast Cancer, I made it my mission to educate the community, young and old, about Inflammatory Breast Cancer (IBC) and ageism. I found that very few breast cancer organizations even mentioned IBC because of its rarity. However, people were interested in the symptoms of Inflammatory Breast Cancer because they were unlike any form of breast cancer they had heard of. I had the opportunity to be featured in two commercials, radio advertisements, Rose Parade Floats, local News Special Reports, Talk Radio, local newspapers, Forbes Magazine, and Oprah Magazine sharing my bout with IBC. Inflammatory Breast Cancer was scary, but someone had to start the conversation and I was okay with being that someone. KSIBCF's awareness began with high school students because IBC is typically found in young adults. By educating teenagers and young adults we planted a nugget that may be worth gold in their future.

The other focus of Kommah Seray Inflammatory Breast Cancer was ensuring patient's survival through treatment. Our programs and services included financial, transportation, and prescription assistance, peer counseling, advocacy, and keeping client's company during treatment. We fundraised and sought out grant funding to keep our clients afloat. KSIBCF was a labor of love on so many levels. It was a volunteer ran organization for the first five years, then after creating sustainable fundraising income streams, we were able to employ Olivia Williams as Coordinator over the Patient Assistance Program and myself as Executive Director. We were changing lives, we were making a difference, and this was my desired legacy.

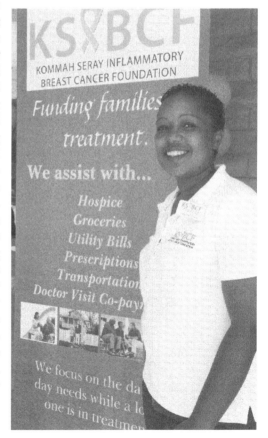

52

Surviving

"Hold your head high, stick your chest out. You can make it. It gets dark sometimes, but morning comes. Keep hope alive."

Jesse Jackson

Six months after radiation treatment ended, while planning for reconstructive surgery, everything came to a screeching halt, *again.* New lumps appeared in my left breast. Not only was this new discovery unnerving, it was also puzzling. Since the study of Inflammatory Breast Cancer was still so limited, there were so many uncertainties as to what to do next. My medical team closely monitored the lumps for an additional six months, and as a team, we decided to remove them as a preventative measure. So, in addition to reconstruction, I was scheduled to have a prophylactic mastectomy (skin sparing mastectomy) in the summer of 2007.

On Monday, July 2, 2007, Dr. Shen performed the skin sparing mastectomy by removing my areola to excise the breast tissue in my left breast and Dr. Tan, my plastic surgeon, and his team performed one of four schedule surgeries, the abdominal trans flap bilateral reconstruction of both breasts. In layman's term, Dr. Tan used the skin and healthy fat from my stomach to reconstruct my right breast and the fat was also used to refill my left breast through my areola. As part of the reconstructive process, my areola and nipples were scheduled to be tattooed on my new breast in the final surgery, which would represent the completion of my breast reconstruction.

Surgery began at 7:00 a.m. and I was in recovery by 11:45 p.m.. Of course, it seemed like five minutes to me, but my mom, husband, and godmother, felt all 16 hours and 45 minutes of the surgery as they sat in the waiting room.

On Tuesday, I woke to see my husband laying at the foot of my bed. He was so glad to see me open my eyes and boy was I glad to see him. He told me surgery went longer than expected, but everything went well, and they didn't want to rush. After a brief conversation, I spent most of the day sleeping off the anesthesia and pain medication. Ministers from my church at the time, St. Stephen Baptist Church, stopped by to check on me, but I was either sleep or too tired to speak.

The following day was 4th of July and we had planned to celebrate our independence in the hospital as I recovered from surgery. My sister visited baring gifts and festive head gear. My mom just loved on me as much as she could while Charles and I were too tired to celebrate due to the nurses monitoring my transferred skin every 15 minutes throughout the night. We learned that the first 48 hours were critical to the survival of the skin when it is transferred to a different part of the body. The nursing team had to keep a close eye to see if my body would accept or reject the transfer. This was a grueling process, but very necessary. Fortunately, my family and I were able to see the fireworks through the window. Once they were done, everyone kissed me goodnight, including my Charles, as they all had to work the next day.

Thursday was a pretty long day for me. I was supposed to be able to eat real food, have visitors, and physical therapy was going to give me a shower and walk me around the room and recovery area. My mom was going to spend time with me before she had to go to work and Sis. Dawkins was scheduled to keep me company for a few hours after my mom left. Then my mother-in-law's hung out with me until Charles could get there… *at least that was the plan for the day.*

Everything seemed to go awry right from the jump. As I attempted to enjoy breakfast, I felt sick very shortly after starting my meal. The nurse had to give me nausea medicine to help keep what little food I ate down. Then physical therapy came to show me how to get up from the hospital bed by using ONLY my leg muscles. This was critical because I needed to move to increase the blood circulation in my legs. Getting up was the hardest thing I had to do. I could not believe how hard it was for me to sit up, stand up, and then walk. I only took a few steps and when the nurse put me back in bed, I needed pain medicine and a nap. I slept until my mom arrived and I woke to her beautiful face. Boy was I glad to see her. I told her about my adventurous day and how I wasn't looking forward to walking again. We then talked and did a little bit of nothing together.

At 9:15 am, my mom left and Sis. Dawkins arrived. She was glad to see I was doing well and looking well. We talked, watched TV, slept, and ate lunch together. I really appreciated her taking the time to sit with me. At about 2:00 p.m., my mother-in-law, Janice McDowell, arrived and Sis. Dawkins tapped out. Mom and I talked a while as she sorted through her stack of bills and other to-do items, which was normal for her. She also was able to witness me having to get up, so I could use the restroom and then getting back into bed. My legs were so extremely sore from the day before because I was not able to use any arm or stomach muscles, so ALL of my weight fell on my legs. Feeling helpless, mom tried to assist where she could, but my thighs were shaking so bad, it was difficult to get them to cooperate, they were tired. With every ounce of mental and physical strength, I was able to relieve myself and get back in bed. Everything hurt, I just prayed for the time to pass and for my legs to hurry up and get use to supporting my body. Who knew using the restroom could be so difficult? Finally, at about 5:30 p.m., my knight in shining armor arrived and he took over from there. He was a little tired but kept me company until about 9:00 p.m. He headed home, as he had an internal interview the next day to prepare for.

On Friday, my doctor gave me the option for an early release from the hospital because I was doing so well. I choose to leave so I could get home to begin my healing process and I was so tired of the beeping machines. In preparation for my discharge, all IVs were removed, and I was able to practice walking a little more. My mom came to stay with me that morning and I received my final lessons on how to shower post-surgery with drains. I was excited, and my recovery was looking great, so far. By the time Charles arrived to take me home, most of the day had passed. He arrived in a good mood because his interview went well, despite how mentally and physically exhausted he was. He was even more excited to learn that I had been discharged and we were leaving the hospital. After a brief training on how to care for me and the drains coming out of my chest, we left.

The ride home was rough. It was hard getting in the car and sitting comfortably. We made it home and I was able to rest in my late grandpa's electric recliner that helped me stand up or lay flat. This amazing piece of furniture was designated as my bed during recovery because of its super powers. My pain levels were manageable; however, there was a mix up with my prescriptions, so we were not able to get them filled. Thankfully, our neighbors came over to visit and brought ice cream. To their surprise, they ended up neighbor-sitting me while Charles went back to City of Hope to get a new prescription and drive across town to the nearest 24-hour pharmacy to fill the prescription. During this time, my neighbors learned very quickly how to help me to the restroom. They were also the first to witness my first cough, which was HORRIFIC!!

I was in soooo much pain, tears began to flow. I thought my stitches were going to burst, the pain was excruciating. Finally, Charles made it back home and he was so tired from running around town that he was done for the day. Shortly after, we prepared for bed. I took my meds, and we figured out the right pillow combination for propping my legs, butt, and head up while I slept. Thankfully, we slept through the night, but that morning was very scary. I took my morning meds and an hour later, I threw them up. We tried a little chicken broth to settle my stomach, but I couldn't keep that down either. By this time the Homecare nurse had called and said she would be there to help us in 90 minutes. Unfortunately, I was in too much pain to wait for her, so we decided to go to Triage at City of Hope. After receiving medicine and being examined to ensure all stitches were intact, we were sent back home. But before leaving, Charles was able to ask some clarifying questions to help us manage things at home. From there we went home to take a nap.

The Home Healthcare nurse came to check on me and was impressed that we knew what to do. We had the drains under control and all bandages were replaced properly. So, just to give Charles a break, she offered to give me fresh dressings for ALL my bandages. Normally this would be well received, but this particular nurse sweated so bad during the process, she was raining sweat all over everything. We were so disgusted by this, Charles had to leave the room to stop himself from laughing in her face. If that wasn't bad enough, once she finished the bandages, her attention turned to my bowel movements. She asked me for the date and time of the last time I had had a bowel movement and I told her, the day before my surgery. After calculating the number of days, her concern intensified. I tried to explain to her that the doctor told me my bowel movements would stop for at least four days while I was on bed rest, then they would gradually start back up again. So, technically, it had only been two days. After much convincing, the nurse accepted my explanation and left for the day.

To our surprise, the next day we were visited by another Home Healthcare nurse. This time, she came running up our driveway waving a box of enemas in the air.

"Hello! I brought an enema for your wife since she is constipated." She yelled.

Apparently, the first nurse shared her concerns about my bowels, so she too was very concerned.

"NO… thank… you!" I said.

I then went on to explain how I was only on the third day after the catheter was removed and I should have a bowel movement by Sunday or Monday. Again, she stressed the importance of the bowel movement and insisted on leaving the enemas behind, just in case. When she finally left, we enjoyed a good laugh at her expense.

Fortunately for me, I did not need an enema. The doctors were right, it happened all on its own. Subsequently, on Monday, Charles and I agreed to cancel the Home Healthcare nurses because they were too intense for us. Charles continued to log my drains volume, discharge, changed bandages, monitored my medicine, scheduled caregivers, helped with physical therapy, monitored my transferred skin, cooked, cleaned, and worked. He had everything under control.

The next day was a big day toward recovery. The fluid buildup was draining as expected, so the doctor removed five of the six drains and left me with one for a little longer. I was glad to be relieved of the five but, that one was still so uncomfortable. Then, at the end of the week, the last drain was pulled out… I was finally detached from everything. I was getting stronger by the day and I was able to walk to my doctor's appointment without my walker, which felt good. I slept for three hours after that appointment, my body was so tired.

The next day, I moved on to the next stage of my recovery and I was introduced to a recovery girdle. I had to wear a tight fitted griddle all day. I didn't like the griddle because it was extremely tight. It also cut off the circulation in my legs because my torso so short. I had to take a pain pill at night because it was so uncomfortable. A few days later, as I was getting in bed, I realized my right breast was much colder than the rest of my body. We were a little concerned, but I attributed this to the griddle being too tight, so we called the triage nurse at City of Hope. We were given the option to go back to Triage to have it checked out. I was tired and didn't feel like going, so we decided to watch the skin through the night and call the doctor in the morning. We woke up a few times and checked for discoloration, per our warning signs instructions, and we checked to see if there was a difference in temperature. By morning, the temperature remained the same, but the skin began bruising. This, of course, was very alarming. I called my plastic surgeon's office and they graciously squeezed me in their schedule. Dr. Tan was a little concerned with the bruising and the redness under the reconstructed right breast. A week later, the bruising started to lighten up and the pigmentation of my skin started to fade. My skin was dying. Charles rushed me back to City of Hope. It was discovered that my griddle was resting too high under my right breast and was affecting the circulation to that area. After trimming the griddle, I was sent home and although the discoloration remained the same, the skin was ok.

Overall, the appearance of the first stage of four reconstructive surgeries was amazing. I had two breasts, which will forever be known as my fraternal twins, unwanted belly fat was excised from my pooch and I had a perfectly sculpted stomach. I often refer to this as my "Tummy Tuck." I was very pleased with the end result, although the recovery was unimaginably difficult.

Recovery from this type of surgery took two months to just sit up straight and stand using my abdominal muscles. My stomach was so tight, I was bent over for the first four weeks. With weeks of physical therapy, I began to straighten out one-month post-surgery. In the second month, I was learning how to reengage my abdomen for sitting, standing, and other basic functions I took for granted. By the end of the second month, I was able to drive and move about independently. Elated to be free, I was mentally gearing up for the next surgery in the reconstructive process. I struggled with the thought of going under the knife again, but since I had already started the process, Charles and I thought it would be best to just get through it.

A few months later, I had the second reconstructive surgery. This surgery was intended to balance things out once the transferred skin was accepted. It was also an opportunity to correct any areas that may have been overlooked or did not heal properly. Unlike the first 16-hour surgery, the second stage only lasted four hours. However, unlike the first surgery, my body had a tough time waking up from the anesthesia. I recall being extremely groggy and not able to speak or see clearly. I felt strange, as if something was wrong. Considering this was my fourth surgery in two years, I was a little unnerved by how I was feeling. So, I asked the nurse about the lingering effects in hopes for some insight that would help put me at peace.

"Sometimes it takes a little longer for your body to wake up, that's all." She answered casually.

Sadly, her words were not comforting to me, I instinctively knew that my body was tired, too tired. After several hours in the recovery unit, I was released to go home. Once home, Charles and I discussed how tired I really felt and that my body had been through enough. I asked Charles if he was okay with my breast being different, his opinion was all that mattered to me. Gratefully, that night we both agreed that I was done with the reconstructive process. This decision did not come easy, especially at a time where body image means so much. I grappled with not being able to wear certain blouses or dresses because my chest wall was compromised. My breasts were not balanced at all and due to the radical mastectomy, which removed all the skin and breast tissue from my right side, I was still slightly concaved after the second surgery. Unfortunately, this imperfection was rather obvious in low cut tops, dresses, and especially bathing suit tops. As I stared at my fraternal twins, I thought, "Can I live with you? Are you enough? Would I ever regret not going any further?"

During my follow-up visit with my reconstruction surgeon, I informed him of our decision to not complete the remaining two surgeries. After much discussion, Dr. Tan respected my decision and continued to monitor me through the complete healing from both surgeries.

"Wow!!" I thought.

I was done with chemo, radiation, and surgeries. I was FINALLY finished!

Advocacy

*Even hope may seem but futile, when with troubles you're
beset, But remember you are facing just what
other men have met.*

Edgar A Guest Trouble

After the completion of my treatment, I was invited to join a newly
established Patient and Family Advisory Council (PFAC) at City of Hope.
This was my opportunity to make a difference in Cancerville, the cancer
world, as a young adult, and to ensure IBC was included in the conversation.
PFAC consisted of City of Hope patients, caregivers, doctors, administrators,
and volunteers. Each member of PFAC played an intricate role in creating a
patient and family centered culture at City of Hope. We used our everyday
experiences to address everyday problems from the various vantage points.
We worked with any and every department that had a desire to gain a patient's
perspective on their day-to-day operations. We tackled any project that
involved a patient and vetted all options prior to providing input. PFAC
taught me that the patient's voice must be heard during their journey through
Cancerville. No two patients were alike, so it was necessary to respect
patient's differences and allow for all voices to be heard.

I learned so much from PFAC that I mirrored its philosophy with
KSIBCF. I became an empowered Patient Advocate that was able to see the
needs of cancer patients and provide supportive resources to help them
through Cancerville. Then, through patient advocacy, I learned about the
Center of Community Alliance for Research and Education (CCARE) at City
of Hope. Under the direction of Dr. Kimlin Ashing, I had the opportunity
to collaborate with CCARE through the African American Breast Cancer
Advocate & Research Coalition on several research projects and academic

publications throughout the years.

CCARE inspired me to pursue additional community collaboratives, which lead to KSIBCF and me individually partnering with City of Hope Patient Navigation and Breast Cancer Study, a Steering Committee Member for OurHope, City of Hope's Rapid Improvement Engagements, Breast & Cervical Cancer Collaborative, Breast Cancer Solutions partnership, Susan G. Komen, American Cancer Society, Living Beauty, Inland Empire Cancer Coalition, Michigan State University and many more local organizations within Cancerville. KSIBCF also participated in the Building Sustainable Community Based Research Infrastructure to Better Science (CRIBS) 2012 Intensive Training Program (ITP), which was a collaboration between the California Breast Cancer Research Program (CBCRP) and Commonwealth. CBCRP is a state funded program administered by the University of California, Office of the President, whose mission was to eliminate breast cancer by leading innovation in research, communication, and collaboration in the California scientific and lay communities.

As the doors began to open; I became a valued member of Cancerville, and I was given several opportunities to be a voice for those who felt they had no voice or were misunderstood by medical professionals. As a Patient Advocate, the voice of the patient, I often sat as a panelist for health-related conferences and trainings. I was a presenter for patient advocacy in collaboration with research studies KSIBCF participated in. I personally represented the patient's voice on doctor's panels and intensive trainings. This path also led me to becoming certified in Professional Advancement in Philanthropy and Protecting Human Research Participants. My arsenal of knowledge, research, and resources was equipping me to make a difference in Cancerville for all who found themselves passing through.

The more I became involved in this community, the more I realized there was a need for the services KSIBCF would offer to patients in treatment. More importantly, I discovered an underserved population of cancer patients, the economically defined *"middle class"*, which became the focus of KSIBCF. I quickly realized, I was middle class. My husband and I made enough money to live comfortably prior to getting cancer. Charles owned a home, had two paid off cars, I had a paid off vacation timeshare, we had established multiple savings accounts, we both had investments, and disposable income. We were DINKies… Double Income, No Kids. We traveled often, as friends and once married. We were comfortable. But, once cancer treatment bills started rolling in, even with insurance, it is like a tsunami overtook our life. Bill after bill rolled in with no end in sight.

As a patient, battling cancer is hard enough on the body, but when you add the pressure of bills and one's inability to work during treatment, it is overwhelming. Furthermore, as caregivers try to manage life, work, and their loved one's treatment schedule, they find it defeating trying to keep up with the revolving bills.

We quickly discovered that many families found themselves wading in the River of Life that flowed through Cancerville. As they attempted to cross the river, they were often forced further and further from stability when bills, insurance, work, family, and friends knocked them over. They tried scurrying to their feet and finding their footing between treatments, only to be crushed by yet another bill. Fortunately for me, on the other side of the river was my support team casting out rafts. With their support, many of our day-to-day needs were met. Sadly, that was not the case for other patients and I wanted KSIBCF to be an organization that would cast out rafts for those in need. It would not discriminate against cancer type, gender, or age. We would serve anyone in need to get them to the other side of treatment.

PFAC also lead me to an amazing opportunity of becoming a patient speaker for City of Hope through the Philanthropy Department. It is there that I discovered my gift of inspirational words, my fuel for advocacy, and the yearning for my legacy to be shared. As I began the speech writing process, I became grateful for the speech class I took many years prior at Covina High School. It was there that I learned how to write various types of speeches; persuasive, informative, and speeches for special occasions. I also learned that the power of any speech is in its delivery. I was taught how to set my voice to the cadence of my message, pause for impact, articulate clearly, accentuate main points appropriately, and adjust my volume flawlessly. As one cursed with facial expression beyond my control, under most circumstances, public speaking was the best platform that allowed my expressions to align with the passion of my thoughts, my voice, my story. For three years, I entered and placed in several high school public speaking contests. I was comfortable on the stage standing before audiences delineating a given topic. Public speaking demanded self-confidence. I struggled with perfectionism in the beginning, but time taught me that no one was perfect and a skilled speaker learned from the blunders in delivery.

Decades later, I traveled the country as a patient speaker, sharing my story of hope to donors and supporters. I shared my story because as a patient of City of Hope, I was afforded the opportunity of a lifetime, LIFE! With God's guidance, my medical team was awesome, and I could not be more pleased with my treatment process. I knew I made the right decision to switch my care to such an esteemed institution where I was confident my doctors had my best interest in mind. Words cannot express how grateful my family and I are for my second chance at life.

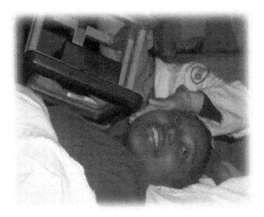

I realize that my outcome is different than the vast majority who do not survive Triple Negative Inflammatory Breast Cancer. My treatment was successful because of researchers and doctors like Dr. Somlo who specialized in the study of Inflammatory Breast Cancer. So, because of my journey with City of Hope, I share my story as a way of thanking them for their role in saving my life.

A Miracle

"Hope deferred makes the heart sick,
but a longing fulfilled is a tree of life."

Proverbs 13:12 (NIV)

In June of 2006, after my last radiation treatment, Charles and I had promised that we would not intentionally get pregnant for two years due to safety concerns. Despite the fact that I was already in menopause from my chemo treatment, we honored this request for exactly two years. Then, almost to the date, my body came out of menopause after 13 months and we decided to stop all precautionary measures. To our surprise, in August of 2008, we discovered I was three months pregnant. Truthfully, in July I had suspected something was going on with my body, but we had planned a trip to our favorite theme park, Magic Mountain, and I wanted to ride all the rollercoasters. So, I kept my inkling to myself until after our trip.

On the last weekend of July, we headed to Magic Mountain to celebrate the birthdays of our nephew, Eligah turning 14 and cousin Tyron, turning 13 years old. Proudly, we were all rollercoaster fanatics, the more dips and flips the better. As we stood in line after line, I read and reread all the warnings posted. "People with the following conditions should NOT ride: Expecting Mothers..." Selfishly, I said a little prayer as I continued to board every ride in the park. I figured, this would be my last rollercoaster for a while, so I should make the most of it. Besides, if I were expecting, I could not have been too far along so there shouldn't be any effect on the baby. I tried everything to justify my selfish decision. It worked, I had a great time and no one knew any different, but when we started heading home, guilt began to weigh on me.

"What have I done? What if I am pregnant? Oh, my goodness, did I just scramble my egg?"

How would I or could I tell Charles, he would be so upset with me for risking our child's life for a rollercoaster ride. What if this was our only shot at getting pregnant? I may have very well compromised our future. Not sure of what to do, I waited a few days before purchasing a pregnancy test. I wasn't too sure how to tell Charles about my inkling because if I were more than a month pregnant, I knew he would put two and two together. But I hoped that he would think I didn't know any better.

I took the test, it was positive... we sat speechless for a few minutes. Our eyes connected and we screamed, hugged, laughed... kissed. Emotions just flooded our bodies. We did it! Without any intervention or even trying, we did it. After confirming the pregnancy with multiple store-bought tests and a blood test, we were so elated, and amazed at what God could do. Statistically, I had a zero percent chance of having a child... *zero!* Charles was so happy, words cannot express how grateful he was to become a father. He told me he knew the Lord would give us a child, it was just a matter of time. We were so excited, yet very nervous too. As much as we wanted to share our news with family and friends, we waited a month longer in fear of a miscarriage or any daunting news that we needed to brace ourselves for. Doctor's ran several tests to see if there were signs of irregularities due to my exposure to chemo and radiation. Fortunately, all was well and it was okay to share the news with family and friends.

Not only were our loved ones excited, my plastic surgeon was relieved because he was concerned about me gaining weight after having the tummy tuck a year prior. I was dieting and working out, but I could not stop the weight from creeping on me. I was so glad to be able to tell my surgeon, Dr. Tan, "I have an excuse for gaining weight, I'm pregnant." We laughed long and hard because he knew how hard I was working to maintain my flat stomach. But, then, after thinking about all I had gone through with that surgery, I was slightly upset because I felt like I was wasting a perfectly good tummy tuck.

Initially, I was considered a high-risk pregnancy, but after months of tests and healthy check-ups, that designation was removed. However, as a breast cancer survivor, I was terrified. I was concerned about the impact chemo would have on my eggs long term. I toiled over the extensive radiation therapy I had to undergo. Although, I must acknowledge the fact that my Radiation Oncologist, Dr. David Wong, from City of Hope took extra precautionary measures in protecting my reproductive organs, *just in case* I was able to get pregnant. I was so grateful he took the time to look beyond my present situation and considered my future, despite the survival statistics.

My pregnancy was flawless, and I was able to carry our son until full-term. A day after my due date, March 28, 2009, I told Charles, "I think I am in labor." Becoming a new dad and nervous, he grabbed the hospital bags, put me in the car and we headed to the hospital. When we arrived at the Birthing Center, I pushed the buzzer for the nurse to let us in. Over the speaker the nurse asked, "Yes, how may I help you?"

"I think I am in labor." I replied very calmly.

"You THINK, you are in labor…" She laughed through the intercom. "Honey, if you were in labor you would KNOW it…" She said.

Then she buzzed us back and put me in a room to be examined. She and all the nurses at the station near our room were laughing at us and eventually we were released to go home to wait a little longer. I was very upset with the nurse for laughing at me. This was my first child, how was I supposed to know when I was in *actual* labor or not? But, before we left the Birthing Wing, another nurse pulled me to the side and gave me a birthing tip.

She told me, "go home and run a bath with water as hot as I could stand it. Then put Epson salt in it. Sit in the bath for at least 30 minutes and that will trigger your contractions."

We drove home from the hospital feeling a little humiliated from being laughed out of the Wing, but I was grateful for the tip. As instructed, I ran a bath with Epson salt and sat in it for 30 minutes. Right before I was done with the bath the contractions hit… one after the other… the pain was indescribable.

I called for Charles and said, "it's time, it's time… I am in labor!"

He quickly helped me out of the bath and dressed me as the contractions began to roll in. He then put me in the car and drove to the hospital as fast as he could, knowing that this time it was for real. When we arrived at the hospital, about four hours after our first visit, I pushed the buzzer to the Birthing Wing.

The nurse on the other end said, "Yes, how may I help you?"

"I AM in labor!" I said very confidently.

When they buzzed me in and saw that I was back, the nurse said, "I told you you would know when you were in labor."

66

I chuckled but was quickly interrupted by a contraction. Now I was able to understand why I was laughed out of the hospital the first time, I couldn't even be mad.

After a few hours of laboring, the pain was too much to bear, so I opted for an epidural. It seemed like it took forever for the doctor to finally make his way to my room to give me some relief. After the epidural, the pain subsided but I was not dilating. The nurse grew very concerned and decided to check if the baby was in the right direction. During her exam, she was able to touch the top of his head, but then he floated back up into my stomach. This was strange and cause for alarm. She then examined the outside of my stomach and asked me if anyone ever considered any complications due to my hip-to-hip scar from my reconstructive surgery? I told her my OB/GYN was aware of my scar, but it was never an issue. The nurse then left the room and returned with a doctor, more nurses and an ultrasound machine. After some discussion, she used the ultrasound machine to look at my hip-to-hip scar, then everyone left the room. The nurse returned with the emergency on-call doctor and after he checked my cervix and confirmed that I was not dilating, he said, "Well, we thought you were going to be here for a while, but your baby can't get past your scar tissue. We have to do an emergency C-section."

"An emergency C-section?" I thought. My nerves were bad enough from having to get the epidural, now this?

Suddenly, the doctor and nurses started moving about the room preparing me for surgery. I was told that I would be awake during the delivery, but I would not feel a thing because of the epidural. Charles and I were relieved because I did not want to experience anymore pain. As promised, the epidural kicked in, but before I knew it, I was out. Sometime later, I woke up in a bright white surgery room and all I could see were people moving around me prepping for the C-section. A few minutes passed, then a nurse saw that I was awake.

She came over with a smile and said, "Hello, Mrs. McDowell. Are you ok?"

"Yes." I replied.

She looked puzzled. "Mrs. McDowell, are you ok?" She said a second time.

"Yes, yes I am ok." I replied.

"Doctor, she isn't responding." The nurse said.

"What do you mean? I am responding. I said I am ok. Why can't you hear me?"

The doctor came into view. "Mrs. McDowell, if you can hear me, move your fingers."

"Ok, I am." I said.

"Mrs. McDowell, if you can hear me, I need you to move your fingers." The doctor said with a stern voice.

"I am, I am moving them…" I yelled.

He then turned to the nurse, "she is not responding."

He turned back to me, "Kommah, I need you to move your fingers if you can hear me."

I began to cry and yelled, "I am, I am… why can't you hear me. What is happening?"

Both the doctor and nurse stepped to the side and all I could hear him say was, "I hate to have to do this, but we don't have a choice."

I began to cry, and I tried with all my might to move something, anything, so that they knew I was alive. The nurse turned around quickly and said, "Oh no, she is panicking. She is having a panic attack."

"I am not panicking, I just want you to know I'm alive, I'm alive." I cried.

The next thing I knew, the nurse walked over with a clear mask that cupped my nose and mouth and said, "I'm sorry."

"Noooo!" I yelled. "Please don't, I am here, I'm alive. Nooooo."

I felt myself slipping away… "Am I dying? What happened? What went wrong… I'm dying…" I was so scared and confused. I didn't know what went wrong or how. After a few seconds, I accepted my fate and I asked for the Lord to forgive me for my sins. Then I thanked God for allowing me to live long enough to give birth to our son. I told God, if my purpose in life was to have a son, then I fulfilled my assignment. I prayed for my family and I started the Lord's Prayer until I was gone...

"Mrs. McDowell…. Mrs. McDowell" A small voice called.

"Is that God?" I thought. "Was I in heaven?" My eyes flew open…

No, it was the nurse trying to wake me up. I couldn't believe it.

I WAS ALIVE.

I was so excited I tried to speak, but nothing would come out. I tried again and again, still nothing. I tried clearing my throat and it hurt so bad, but I had to speak, so I tried once again, and an audible sound came out. The nurse turned and looked at me.

"Are you trying to speak?" She asked. "You have had a long night, try to get some rest."

I tried again, with everything I had, "Did I die?" I asked.

"What, what are you trying to say? They had to put a breathing tube in your mouth, so your throat will be sore for a while. Just rest."

"Did I die?" I asked again. This time she was able to make out my words.

"Did you die? Are you serious? Mrs. McDowell, please just get some rest. You obviously are very tired."

I was so confused and too afraid to close my eyes. I laid in the recovery room refusing to rest, finally my mom was allowed to come see me. When she entered the room ready to congratulate me, I began to weep, and I held her so tight. I told her that I thought I died during the surgery and they must have resuscitated me. She was so confused about what I was saying, so she just rocked me until I was able to gain my composure.

I asked, "Where is Charles, where is my baby?" She told me that they were in the nursery waiting for me to come out of recovery. Apparently, I had been in recovery for over four hour and it was after 11:00 p.m. at night. My godmother then came in to report that I instructed Charles to stay with the baby, no matter what, so he has been standing next to him the entire time. He was tired and after the third hour he sat on the floor by the bassinet, where he still was. He had not eaten or gone to the restroom in four hours. She also told me that Charles hadn't even held his son yet because he wanted me to be the first person to touch him. I was so overwhelmed by how amazing my husband was. He honored my request to stay with the baby when I knew his heart was longing for me.

Finally, 30 minutes later, I was wheeled into a private room. Immediately after the nurse cleared me, Charles entered the room pushing the baby in the bassinet. He gave me a kiss and a big hug.

"There is someone who would like to meet you face-to-face." He said. Then he pushed the bassinet over and in a soft voice, "Christian, your mommy is ready for you now."

I sobbed and sobbed. Unfortunately, Charles had no idea of the trauma I experienced during the surgery because he was waiting outside. So, he was taken aback by my reaction to both him and Christian. I took my time looking Christian over from head to toe as tears ran down my face. I was so glad to be able to hold him, kiss him, see him. Then, after a few minutes, Charles asked if he could hold his son. I smiled and gently handed him over.

"Thank you, Lord." I thought, "For blessing us with a son." We were so grateful.

After a few minutes, Charles handed Christian back to me and left to tell those family and friends who were still there, that they could visit with us one at a time. My sister was the first person to visit. She entered the room excited and bubbly until she saw my face. Her bubble busted, she immediately ran over and asked, "What's wrong, sissy?"

"I think I died during delivery and they had to bring me back." I told her.

"What?" She said. "Why do you think that?"

I told her what I remember happening and the last thing I remember was me slipping away. "I died." I said as I sobbed.

"It's okay sissy, you are here now, that's all that matters." She held me tight. She then picked up Christian for a few minutes and left the room in tears.

Next, Christian's godparents, John and Maddie Apiafi, entered the room. Fortunately, my sister had warned them about my emotional state of being, so they entered very concerned about me. They asked what happened and I told them what I thought had happened during delivery. Again, I found myself in tears. After trying to console me and saying hello to Christian, they said their goodbyes.

Eventually, everyone went home and Charles, Christian and I were left to rest in our room. Still too afraid to close my eyes, I watched my boys sleep so peacefully. At about 2:00 am, a nurse stopped in to check on us and found me wide awake.

"Why aren't you sleeping?" She asked.

"I am afraid to close my eyes because I think I died during my C-section and they had to resuscitate me." I said as I began to weep again.

"Oh no, sweetie," she said, "I was in the operating room for your delivery, you did not die. You had a panic attack, so we had to put you to sleep."

"I wasn't panicking." I told her, "I was trying to respond but no one could hear me."

"I'm so sorry," she said. "You started thrashing around on the table and we thought you were panicking." "But you were never in any danger."

I was so glad to hear this and I thanked God that she was in the operating room to witness what actually happened. Finally, I was at peace, which allowed me to go to sleep.

For months, I was haunted by this experience, but it made me really appreciate life. This was the second time in my life when I thought I was dying and both times I had to reconcile within myself that this was it. I said my last prayer and gave myself to the Lord. In both instances, I was surprised to wake up, to still be alive. I have learned to be so grateful for the little things in life and I literally live each day like it is my last. Both cancer and child birth were life altering experiences for me and my family.

We were so excited to take our son home, but I was still afraid that he would have side effects from my cancer treatment. Almost immediately, our concerns of treatment side effects grew because he was very gassy and cranky. We learned two things that night. One, Christian was lactose intolerant so we had to switch his formula accordingly. Due to my breast surgeries, my fraternal twins were not capable of nursing him, so we were completely dependent on formula. Secondly, we learned that navigating the world with a newborn was going to be scary at times, and we weren't doing ourselves any favors by automatically assuming my treatment had anything to do with our son crying. Maintaining this mindset was critical to my psyche throughout the years.

At only two weeks old, we noticed bumps all over Christian's little feet. He would rub them together and just cry. After consulting his pediatrician, we discovered he had eczema. "What next?" I thought. I prayed constantly over him, I was so nervous. Then, after about three months, and several visits to the pediatrician, my nerves began to subside, and I started to enjoy motherhood. I had to stop living in fear.

Charles' Perspective

"Faith and hope work hand in hand, however while hope focuses on the future, faith focuses on the now."

David Odunaiya, How To Make Faith Work In Your Life

My journey through cancer and Cancerville was passionately supported by my Charles. So, I would be remiss if I did not take a moment to allow Charles to weigh in on some key moments along the way.

After Koko's initial biopsy, those two days of the Unknown were very worrisome. How do you save face, knowing there is a possibility the one you love may have cancer? I prayed and hoped the surgeon was wrong for two days. Then, on the third day, we went in for the results. As Koko was called from the waiting area and we were ushered to the waiting room, my heart pounded. We were moved several times and the wait seemed like forever.

"We wanted to put you in a more comfortable room while you wait, as the Doctor is clearing a few things to spend more time with you." The nurse commented during one of the moves.

"Why would the Dr· need to spend more time with us if nothing was wrong?" I thought·

Time seemed to go even slower, I was agonizing for the doctor to just come in and say what he needed to say so we could deal with it and move on· Then, finally, after an hour or so, the doctor entered our room and quickly examined Koko·

"You have cancer, two of the three masses we removed were cancerous·" He said with a down cast expression·

There are certain moments in your life you never forget, for me, this was one of those moments· For two days, Koko's mom and I sat silently hoping and praying this would not be the case, but sadly it was· When those words came out of the doctor's mouth, I saw my Koko shed a tear and that broke my heart· Koko is a strong woman and very rarely cried· As expected, each journey of our life together allows us to see different sides of each other· This moment, allowed me to see the vulnerable side of Koko I had not seen before· In my mind, I thought, "What does this mean?" Because all of the people I had known with cancer had died, so I found it difficult to process what the results meant for us and our future· Did it mean the woman I'm willing to give my all to isn't going to be here...What!

I knew I needed to be strong for Koko, so I refuse to sob in front of her, fortunately, I was able to just shed a tear and hold in the flood. After the meeting with the doctor, we walked to our cars in what felt like slow motion. Thankfully, I met Koko and her mom at the doctor's office, so I was able to drive home alone. I was so relieved, because I balled my eyes out. I cried so hard, I'm not even sure how I made it home between wiping my eyes and shifting gears. When we got around the corner from her mom's house, I told myself to get it together. I stopped crying because I needed to present myself as being strong before I enter the house.

I am so glad Koko requested a second opinion, because City of Hope (COH) was a great relief compared to our previous experience with her doctors. Not knowing what to expect, Koko and I appreciated how everyone told us the truth by giving us the hard facts about her type of cancer. The doctors informed us that Koko had a rare form of breast cancer called Inflammatory Breast Cancer (IBC). IBC invades the skin and moves rapidly. With that news, the oncologist wanted to start immediate treatment. They gave us the facts and presented a game plan, which allowed us to deal with our reality without sugar coating it. As a professional trainer, presentation is everything and the way they presented her prognosis was warm and considerate. This was something both of us could deal with, a plan of action.

The game plan began immediately, as Koko needed to have a bone scan, heart scan, chest x-ray, CT scan,

PET scan, and surgery for a port-a-cath. City of Hope had scheduled her chemotherapy for the next 6 months, in hopes to kill and control the rapidly growing cancer cells. After that, she was schedule to have a radical mastectomy, three months of radiation, possible chemo again, and finally, 9-12 months later reconstruction. The doctors were very thorough and when we asked how the treatment process would affect our desires to have children, we were told our chances of having children were slim to none. This hit me pretty hard, I was rendered speechless. As usual, I needed to collect my thoughts and pray.

As our day ended, I recall Koko and I having a heart to heart conversation regarding her diagnosis, the upcoming journey, and slim chances of us having kids. It seemed as though she was trying to give me a get out of jail free pass. I clearly let her know, I was not going anywhere! I didn't wait nearly 30 years to find the woman of my life to just leave. The Bible says, "He who finds a wife, finds a good thing." I prayed and waited for the Lord to send me my good thing and there was no way I was going to let my good thing get away that easily. Ironically, after so many restless nights, that particular night, I slept very well with a sense of unexplainable peace. However, the very next day, we received news that a young adult, who used to attend our church, had just died from Inflammatory Breast Cancer. This was a huge blow to our moral, but since I did not know the lady, I had to help us regain our focus.

"This is just a distraction, we have got to stay focused, everyone is different." I told the family.

Later, I was reminded of God's promise to me. A promise in which I would need to refer to and hang on to for the next three years. I believe God gives us what we need to make it through life, if we just pay attention. This was the first moment in which God prepared me for something prior to my need to understand why. I shared with Koko the promise God had given me, which was my hope for our family. We just needed City of Hope to do their part and God would do the rest.

***

KOKO'S HAIR LOSS

Most of the women in my family had long hair and I've always been attracted to the like. Koko and I, were platonic friends from church for quite a while, but I recall, approximately four years into our friendship, the moment I saw her in a different light. It was at church during a Women's Day concert. She was in the choir stand and had on a white long skirt suit, which was expected, but the way her hair gracefully framing her face combined with her radiant smile, it was like something out of a movie where all I could see was her in the room.

I caught myself thinking, "Wow! Koko looks really

beautiful in that choir stand." Then, I thought, "Why am I thinking this, we are good friends, just friends."

But I couldn't shake it and to this day, that memory never left me because that was the moment, she caught my eye.

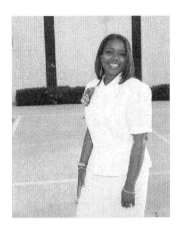

After our engagement, I recall having two dreams about Koko cutting her hair off before our wedding. I didn't think much of the dreams, but considering when I met Koko, she had an afro. So, just to be certain, one day I asked.

"Do you plan on cutting your hair off once we get married?"

I thought maybe she was going to pull the old bait and switch on me.

"No, I don't plan on it." Her response was very nonchalant.

With that, I let it go but I couldn't forget those

dreams. In retrospect, this was the second time I realized God was giving me what I need to make it through. During our meeting with the oncologist at City of Hope, he told us Koko might lose her hair due to the side effect for the type of chemo she needed. I immediately had a flashback to my dreams. Koko became fidgety at this point, because she knew how much I loved her hair. After the meeting she asked me about the possibility of her losing her hair, and I reminded her of the dreams I had had. Little did I know, God was preparing me for this moment and hair loss was the least of our issues, it's just hair. Her hair was what caught my attention, but her heart is what kept it. I have to say, once Koko was bald, she was sexy as ever, her bald head brought more attention to her eyes and cheek bones and I loved it.

***

MANAGING TREATMENT

Being a man of structure and organization, when the doctors told us we needed to devise a plan for managing all appointments, medicines, surgeries, infusions, and check-ups, he was speaking my language. Fortunately, in organizing everything, I realized I could only do so much and we were going to need some serious helping hands. With this reality, when people said, "Let me know what I can do for you," Koko and I did. Because of my work schedule, I wasn't always available to take Koko to and from treatments, therefore, I had to entrust my fiancé/wife to others in my absence.

We were so grateful for our church family, as they were crucial in this process. We were not afraid to ask for help, which allowed us to schedule volunteers around the clock. I created a schedule that included:

- Driving to treatment:
- Driving from treatment:
- Friday shots:
- Company during treatment
    - Person 1:
    - Person 2:
- Company at home
    - Person 1:
    - Person 2:
- Meal deliveries
- Food prep
- Clinic visits
- Visitation days and times

The schedule was quite intricate, because I had to overlap each block of time to account for any delays, changes, or possible emergencies for Koko. Being the person that I am, I would call and email everyone on the schedule each week.

Those looking from the outside may have thought this was a lot of work for me, but I learned in life, you can't put a price tag on a peace of mind.

Fortunately, organization is a natural gift for me and knowing my Koko was in good hands was worth it. This schedule was important for both of us, it provided us with a sense of peace and it was critical to know who was doing what and when. I was able to go to work knowing Koko was in good hands because I knew who to call when I needed to check-in.

***

BODY IMAGE

During this time, I realized the importance of God's word and why purity until marriage was important. I found myself tested in this area from a year prior to dating Koko through our engagement. Maintaining my purity allowed me to get my hormones under control, especially considering Koko's health condition. But finally, on our honeymoon, I was able to let go in a way God intended. It was awesome! But my reality was, access would be very limited for a few years. Therefore, we indulged as much as possible during our three-day honeymoon, but when it was over, we headed home and back into chemo treatments. Because of the rigors of treatment, Koko and I found time for each other after the treatment side effects subsided, approximately day 12 of 14. This was our "normal". I was so grateful when chemo came to an end and surgery was the next phase. Mentally, I figured chemo was the worst part and surgery would be an easier phase to endure.

The surgery phase was easier in the beginning, but her side effects lasted a lifetime, which was nothing I could have imagined. Being merely human, I couldn't foresee the long-term effects so many surgeries would have on my wife. Koko was a strong woman with confidence and strength, but the scars and side effects took some of her spark away. I could see it, but I didn't understand the magnitude of the after-effects until she opened up and we were able to have the hard conversations. She shared with me what her godmother had told her about intimacy. "Wow!" I thought. I was so grateful for that advice. It wasn't ideal, but it was enough to sustain us, considering Koko's reality.

I found myself praying a lot, asking God to restore what we had, to provide wisdom and to send me someone I could talk to. Sadly, in my experience married couples (men) did not discuss their intimacy issues with others. Understanding silence could be a death sentence, God answered my prayer by revealing to me a trusted friend, Brenden McMillan. I recall reaching out to him and sharing my thoughts and feelings regarding intimacy with Koko. I was embarrassed for me and my wife, as Brenden and his wife, Nastashia, were our friends, but this conversation was pushing us to a new level of friendship. After sharing our challenges, Brenden's response was just what I needed.

"Thank you for trusting me and you can be assured I

will not tell anyone·" He said· He went on to say, "Start over, from the beginning· Take the time to explore with touch, gentleness, and talk during the process· You need to communicate, communicate, communicate and rediscover the wife God has sent you·"

His words of wisdom gave me a few golden nuggets to hold on to· He assured me, "It will not happen overnight, but I'm prayerful it will help and please know I will be praying for you and Koko·" His words of wisdom launched a new journey of intimacy as we knew it· Even today, I have not forgotten his words of wisdom and when God provides me with an opportunity to share this with other men, I do· Think about it, this strategy doesn't just apply to illness, it transcends into various aspects of marriage·

***

SURVIVING

Surgery – Oh I hated surgery days· I would find myself very anxious days prior all the way up to the moment Koko was in recovery· I didn't think I could take it anymore, although I never shared that with Koko· My fear was, my Koko wouldn't survive the surgery· We had known a few people who went in for a routine procedure and never woke up from the anesthesia· That, I couldn't deal with· During the second surgery to reconstruct Koko's breast, I was as good as gone· Although, the first 18-hour surgery and recovery time was brutal for me, the second surgery of four hours was a nice change, but no less worrisome. After that surgery, we met with Dr. Tan and he shared the remaining phases of the reconstruction process. It included some clean-up work and nipple tattoos. I recall thinking, "Who needs tattoos, they aren't going to do anything. Besides, I should be the only one seeing them, it's not necessary." But, I felt it was Koko's decision to make. To my surprise, Koko wanted to discuss her reconstruction surgery line up with me and she too had her own set of reservations. Gratefully, Koko and I agreed the next two surgeries were not necessary for us. I could live with her fraternal twins without tattoos, so long as she was here with me. I feared she wouldn't make it out of the next two surgeries and for what... Having my Koko was more important than decorated boobs on a dead wife.

***

A MIRACLE IN THE MAKING

Chemotherapy caused Koko's body to go into menopause when she was only 29 years old. This was one of the side effects discussed prior to treatment, so we were expecting it. Unfortunately, no one knew if her body would revert back to normal after treatment. Fortunately for us, 13 months after treatment, Koko's body began reverting back, but her cycles were inconsistent. There were a couple instances in which we thought she was pregnant, but a few days later aunt flow would arrive. After the second false alarm, I remember saying to myself, "Next time we'll have to wait longer, because in due time, her body will let us know." Remembering what the doctor said, knowing what the reports said, not accepting what the statistics said, I was still holding on to my promise from God, this was my test of faith.

Then, in August 2008, Koko told me, "I think I'm pregnant, I waited longer than normal, and it's been a little while now so I bought another pregnancy test."

She seemed hopeful and antsy as she held up a pregnancy test. She took the test and we waited... 5 min later, the test read positive.

"Wait, what, is that accurate?" I thought, but dare not say out loud.

Excited, yet still skeptical, we scheduled an appointment with the doctor a few days later. It was then that it was confirmed, we were having a baby. My promise has been fulfilled; we were going to have a child.

Koko's pregnancy was flawless. She was closely monitored during the first trimester, but after no signs of concerns, she was considered to have a normal pregnancy. This was a relief to both of us as we prepared for our son's arrival.

Like many couples, we had expected Koko to have a natural child birth, possibly with an epidural, but that was not the case at all. When she went into labor, the medical team ended up wheeling her away to prepare her for an emergency C-section. The nurses told me I could be in the operating room during the procedure, so I was instructed to wait for them to come and get me. Prior to entering the operating room, a nurse explained what was to take place, but circumstances had slightly changed.

"Mr. McDowell, we had to knock Mrs. McDowell out because she began to panic. She when you go in, it will be as we discussed, but she will not be responsive, ok?" The nurse explained.

"Ok!" I said, with no reservation and we headed into the operating room.

Christian was born, and I was given the opportunity to cut his umbilical cord. They cleaned Christian up and I was told I could stay with my wife in recovery. I respectfully declined their offer and I requested to stay with our son. You see, weeks prior, Koko and I had agreed that I would stay with our son, due to the rapid occurrence of baby kidnappings and swaps in delivery wards during that time. Koko had made me promise that I would stay with Christian, NO MATTER WHAT!

Balance

Every day I turn to the Bible to give me strength and wisdom for the day and hope for the future.

Billy Graham

Now as a wife, mother, Executive Director of KSIBCF, community partner, patient advocate, and patient speaker, I had to regain work-life balance. I no longer had the flexibility of coming and going so freely. The foundation was growing, I was traveling to speak more often, I was invited to participate on more panels, gave more presentations, help more patients, and be more involved in the community. All the while, Christian was growing so fast and the depth of my relationship with my husband was growing. Sadly, I was juggling too many responsibilities, hoping to not drop any of them.

As a local advocate in Covina, CA, through KSIBCF, I fought for financial support for families in treatment. Sadly, there are so many charities that claim to support cancer patients, but all they did was provide information and support groups before, during, and/or after treatment. Although these services are necessary, they didn't put food on the table nor did they keep a roof over patient's heads. One of the greatest challenges I faced as Executive Director, was the complete disregard of cancer patient's financial wellbeing during treatment. The clients that sought out KSIBCF were individuals who were having to choose between paying for treatment or paying their bills. Those with children, which encompassed the majority of our clients, juggled treatment, bills, lunches, clothing, supplies and more. My staff and I found ourselves in a role similar to Social Workers. We were working tirelessly trying to help families keep up with life.

Once entrenched in Cancerville, I found that KSIBCF only had a few local allies who were fighting the same fight of not just surviving treatment, but surviving life during treatment. Breast Cancer Solutions, Triple Step for the Cure, Breast Cancer Angels, and Michelle's Place, to name a few. These organizations are still a strong force in the fight of survival today and they cover patients in multiple regions of southern California. Sadly, the needs were and still are great! But the funding was and still is scarce.

Unfortunately, KSIBCF struggled with securing large grant funding that allowed for direct support to patients. However, it was not due to lack of effort, rather grantor's fear of misappropriation of funds. A few years prior to establishing KSIBCF, a handful of non-profits on the national stage found themselves under investigation for fraudulent use of donor dollars. This made it difficult for grassroot organizations, like KSIBCF, to secure funding that did not produce a tangible product. It is with this reality that my perspective of fundraising for KSIBCF changed. We were required to have more sustainable income streams that we could rely on from year-to-year. This gave birth to employee giving campaigns, community awareness walks, merchandise sales, annual galas and so much more. Something had to change, someone needed to represent those who were not able to represent themselves.

KSIBCF began hosting fundraising events for our clients. We shared their stories, their struggles. Just as I had leveraged my story for City of Hope, I found myself asking my clients to do the same for KSIBCF. People needed to know that supporting KSIBCF literally was saving people's lives. Not just poor people either. Unexpectedly, I found that several of our clients were well-to-do prior to treatment bills raining down on them. Clients were spending their life savings just to survive, which ironically, runs out much quicker than it takes to save it. Some clients mortgaged their homes, sold cars, and emptied their children's college funds to survive. Sadly, I was often told that that was the right thing to do. Patients were expected to liquidate all possible accounts and sell all personal property to get through treatment. This mindset infuriated me personally, because I too had to figure out how to survive treatment without losing everything I had worked for, JUST IN CASE I survived. Liquidation was NOT the answer. If I would have liquidated all my assets during treatment, I would have been worse off. What grantors did not understand was, patients who go the route of liquidation find themselves living with people, family or friends. Often times they become a burden, which adds to the existing stressors they are already bearing. Not to mention, patients can be denied treatment if their home environment is not stable or sanitary. Chemotherapy obliterates the immune system, so a patient's living environment is highly critical to their survival.

When I was undergoing chemo, I was told I needed to be quarantined at home the first few days after each treatment. Although I was given an injection to increase my white blood cells after every treatment, it took a few days for my body to produce enough white cells to ward off any bad germs. So, Charles limited my visitor's list down to just a few people. He also made sure everyone washed their hands or used hand sanitizer before entering my room. I had a designated bathroom that was off limits to everyone else. My clothes and sheets were washed a certain way. My food was prepped and cleaned a certain way. Extra precautions were taken to create an environment that minimized any threat to me. We quickly learned it was the little things that counted the most during my journey. We realized, the minor adjustments we made in every aspect of my life were critical to my survival; they were things that went beyond what any pamphlet told us. With this firsthand knowledge, there was so much work to be done in ripping the veil and exposing the critical needs of cancer patients and their families.

This was my fight, and with my allies, we were making headway. We were fighting to illuminate the disparities of individualized care for cancer patients in the service arena. This fight was all-consuming, it required me to leverage the agenda of KSIBCF, raise the awareness of community partners, intensify my patient advocacy, and be the voice for the weary. For four years, I was able to manage all my responsibilities, or so I thought, until one day when I was running out to a meeting. As normal, I called Christian to me and asked for a kiss goodbye.

"Where are you going, mommy?" He asked.

"Mommy has a meeting I have to go to, I will be back soon." I said.

With his big beautiful eyes, he looked at me, paused and said, "Another meeting, mommy?"

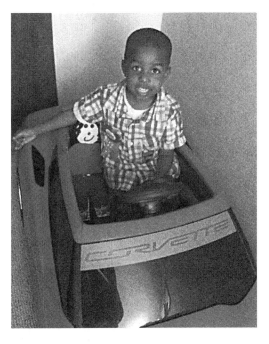

I paused, and at that moment I realized I had dropped one of my responsibilities, my son's heart. In the mist of my hustle and bustle, my son saw the back of my head more than he saw my face. I knew there was a lot wrong with this. I was so busy trying to create a legacy for myself that I didn't realize, he was my legacy. Statistically speaking, I had already surpassed the survival rate for Inflammatory Breast Cancer by four years. I was no longer trying to beat the dooms day clock of two years.

As I ran out for my meeting, I couldn't help but hear his little voice in my head over and over again. He was right. Although I loved the work I did and the people we were able to help, it was all consuming. When I arrived to my meeting, I looked around the table and realized that I was the only young adult in the room with a small child. As a matter of fact, in most of the meetings and groups I attended, I was the only one with a small child. Everyone else either had adult children or no children. I quickly understood that things had to change. I was a mother first, and everything else had to wait. After much prayer and discussion with Charles, we decided it was time to shift our focus from KSIBCF to our family. This meant I had to step down from all other obligations as well. KSIBCF began as a legacy project for my family and friends to carry on in my absence. Ultimately, it turned into my life mission. Sadly, I had to dissolve the organization because it carried my name. The board of directors considered a name change, but we all agreed it would be quicker to simply dissolve the organization.

KSIBCF was blessed to have had amazing board members and advisory board members during its tenure. Past board members consisted of LaNita Odom, Larry Fonville, and Deborah Barber, M.Ed. Past Advisory Board Members consisted of Dr. George Somlo, M.D., F.A.C.P., Oncologist and Director of Breast and Oncology and High-Dose Therapeutics at the time, Jennifer Wendell, Esq. of Carter Wendell Law offices, Zenna Morris, CMF, owner of Sheer Pleasures Boutique that specialized modified garments for breast cancer patients. Kimlin Ashing, Ph.D. of City of Hope, Professor and Director of the Center of Community Alliance for Research and Education, Cathy Cole, R.N.C., N.P., M.P.H., of City of Hope, Clinical Nurse Manager in the Women's Center at the time. Finally, Belinda Torrez, OTR/L. CLT of City of Hope, Rehabilitation Department. Fortunately, I was able to serve as the Executive Director from the beginning to the end.

I recognized that I had a zero percent chance of having a child and the Lord blessed us with Christian. I knew he was not given to us to be forsaken. I choose our son over my career. Many did not understand why I took drastic steps, but I know who I am and how I am. I had to severe my ties with Cancerville or I would be easily drawn back in, it was like an addiction. So, to help make the transition easier for me, we moved to Oceanside, CA, 80 miles away. We wanted a fresh start in a new place where we could raise our son and I could be more available for our family. With great joy, I became a Domestic Engineer.

Labor of Love

"You cannot change anyone but yourself. Always hope for the best, but keep living your life no matter what."

Kate Anderson, 100 Positive Morning Thoughts

Christian was entering kindergarten, as a result, most of my day was spent home alone. We quickly learned that I about lost my mind staying home cooking, cleaning, not interacting with people. I found myself depressed a few months into this new life style. I couldn't handle being cooped up in the house. I needed people, conversation, a social network. So, Charles and I agreed that my time would be better spent volunteering at Christian's school. Fortunately, Christian's teacher, Mrs. Lyndsey Morningstar, welcomed me with open arms. She was only in her second year of teaching, so an extra pair of hands was perfect for her. With her permission, I was able to sashay between being a domestic engineer and a parent volunteer. This allowed me to redirect my itch of serving others through KSIBCF, to volunteering in the classroom and meeting the needs of five- and six-year olds.

This shift was quite interesting in so many ways. I felt as if kindergarteners shared similar issues as adults and I was able to relate to their needs more than I could have ever imagined. They struggled with communicating effectively because of their undeveloped palettes, lack of understanding, or missing teeth. They fought to have their voice heard and their opinion considered in any activity that they were involved in. They were happy to please, some days, and cooperated well other days. Some were confident in their abilities, even at such young ages, while others were very insecure. Many were driven to learn as much as they could, they were like sponges soaking it all up. Yet, others were more apathetic and waited to be told what to do step-by-step. I realized my mother was right after all, children are just little people with the same issues as adults, but with less severe consequences for their actions.

So, after being cleared by the school district and school, I was a regular parent volunteer. Before I knew it, I was in the classroom three to four days a week, helping in any and every way possible. I felt invigorated by helping and Mrs. Morningstar appreciated the support. Before long, she was not able to keep me busy, I was too available, so I began to lend my services to the other Kinder teachers. By the time we reached the third month of school, my face was a regular around campus. I made copies, helped where needed in class, read with students, assisted with art projects, attended all special events, and chaperoned field trips. I loved my new life and I felt fulfilled, I loved the students and the teachers.

During the course of my volunteering, I began to probe teachers, staff and parents about the school's PTA. As a child, my mom was a member of PTA and she enjoyed volunteering at my school. I loved seeing my mom on campus when she was available, it gave me a since of security and it showed me that she cared about me. I remember saying as a child that I was going to be the PTA President when I grew up. Now, decades later, my childhood spark was reignited. Knowing how I have a tendency to be consumed by projects, I was afraid of jumping into something I was not familiar with. I began researching what PTAs did, how they were organized, who they were accountable to, etc. I was surprised to learn that California State PTA governed local school PTAs and that each unit was a subordinate nonprofit organization. As one who loves order and structure, this information excited me and gave me even more reasons to want to get more involved, eventually. I had firsthand experience and knowledge of running a nonprofit organization. This was perfect.

I continued volunteering at the school, now lending my assistance to any teacher or administrator who had a need. I was at school five days out of the week from beginning to end. I missed Cancerville and those I left behind, but volunteering at school helped me to see I could serve anywhere. By the end of the school year, I had made friends with the lower grade kiddos and I loved to hear their little voices call out, "Hi, Mrs. Koko!" It melted my heart, they were worth every minute of my time. Parents began to call me by name, thanks to their son or daughter pointing me out. More importantly, Christian loved to see me around school. Fortunately, he was independent enough to make friends and not hover under me. This was becoming our community and I felt like we belonged.

I then joined PTA, after being approached by Attiyya Ingram and Jeannie

Rogers. They quickly introduced themselves and proceeded to tell me that they had noticed me volunteering around campus. They went on to say that they were the new PTA board for our school and they were recruiting members to help with the upcoming 2015-2016 school year. In my head I thought, "I can't believe they found me, how did they find me? Did someone tell them I was probing? What made them stop me?" Attiyya went on to tell me that she was the incoming President and Jeannie was the Treasurer and they were on a mission to recruit new parents. Then, they asked if I would be interested in the position of Vice President of Ways and Means. I had no idea what that even meant.

"What does a VP of Ways and Means do?" I asked.

"Fundraising, VP of Fundraising." Jeannie said.

"Fundraising, WOW! That is something I know how to do. Let me talk to my husband and I will let you know by the end of the week."

"Okay!" They said.

I walked into the school to my regular scheduled volunteer post. I thought about my encounter all day. I was excited and scared all at the same time. I didn't know if I was ready to jump into PTA just yet, but I couldn't wait to get home to tell Charles.

After much discussion with my husband, we agreed that it was a good time to become more involved in our community. I gladly accepted the Vice President of Ways and Means position. I was confident in my new role, although it officially began in a few months. For nine years, all I did was fundraising for KSIBCF. I had learned a thing or two about raising money and I knew this task would be even easier since I had a captive audience, the kids. "Wow, what an opportunity," I thought.

I saw PTA as a wonderful way to serve students, teachers, and parents. Over the course of three school years, and under the direction of the Principal, I served as VP of Ways and Means, President, and Executive Vice President, in that order.. As a skilled fundraiser, I knew we would be able to raise enough money to meet any pressing needs of the school. I was willing to lend my professional skills to this organization and devote my time and energy to ensuring its success. I worked 40 to 60 hours a week, all three years, serving my community. I believed in unifying people and inclusion, therefore, I organized committees for everything. People who had a desire to volunteer in any capacity were able to do just that, big or small, we took them all. As a team, we found creative ways to raise funds, while only hosting one major fundraiser a year. This methodology worked well and we were able to raise over $285,000 within my three-year span of service. Our unit was strong and effective. We were able to meet and exceed the needs of the students, teachers, and school.

All of my time and energy was poured into my volunteerism. My family sacrifice was significant, but they were willing to share and assist when needed. As expected, I lived and breathed PTA, I was fully consumed. I saw this as an opportunity to leave a footprint on the lives of so many children. I laughed, cried, danced, played, and corrected in love. Often times, parents asked me why I did what I did for our school. My reply was and still is, I have the opportunity to make a difference in the lives of so many little people. Every day, I try to breathe life into who they are and who they want to become. I listen to the kids and I respect them as little people whose opinions, feelings, and presences matters. I embrace their idiosyncrasies that often times drives other adults crazy. I let them be who they truly are and I find ways to hone their positive attributes and redirect their negative ones. Now, understand, I demand respect from every child, but I also give respect to every child. I make it clear that I am not their friend, but I am a trusted adult who hears and sees them. This matters, they matter.

My desire was to inspire the future of our country to be the best people they could be. To inspire a generation to believe in themselves and to use unfortunate life events as a launching pad for something great to come. This was why I was willing to give my all to PTA and volunteering in classrooms. One would be amazed at the brilliant minds we are surrounded by in an elementary school. I know so many parents who wish they were able to be more involved in their children's life, but are unable to for many reasons. I didn't take this opportunity for granted and I was willing to place my life on pause for the sake of my child and the children around me.

For three years, I danced, laughed, played, talked to, heard, and loved on the students. As life would have it, I transitioned from volunteering my time to becoming a substitute teacher. Now, I am able to serve in a different capacity. After only a few weeks of subbing, I realized that my opportunity for impact was even greater in the classroom. I take subbing seriously and by no means am I a glorified babysitter. My expectations for students match that of their teachers. I work hard to ensure students are learning and growing intellectually and socially. I am grateful for my PTA days, because I have established a rapport with students that transcends into the classroom. I respect each student and in return, they respect me. I love subbing!

Reflection

In fact, hope is best gained after defeat and failure, because then inner strength and toughness is produced.

Fritz Knapp, Vince Lombardi: Toughness

In July 2018, I celebrated 13 years of survival. After celebrating 13 years, you would think I should have a peace of mind by now. My life was great. I felt great, I was a domestic engineer most days, but my superhero alias was a substitute teacher. Sadly, peace of mind was far from my reality. I struggled often with the thought of cancer returning. I have prayed many nights that I would remain cancer free. When working KSIBCF, I was faced with assisting clients who were on their second or third bout with cancer. If that wasn't scary enough, I had a friend who was a six-time breast cancer survivor and none of them were a reoccurrence. I became paranoid from time to time and found myself requesting full body scans more often than required. As hard as I tried not to project my clients' diagnosis on myself, I did. Mentally, I carried a fear of the unknown that I could not overcome.

After years of helping others through treatment, I realized I was still too close to my client base. I had not had enough time or distance from my journey to be able to see each client's journey as their own. I was beginning to have restless nights and was becoming emotionally attached to clients. Finally, I had to come to terms with the fact that I was human, and I too could have benefited from the services KSIBCF offered.

By starting KSIBCF immediately after my treatment ended, I did not allow myself time to heal mentally and emotionally from wading in the waters of Cancerville, raft or no raft. I didn't recognize that my journey was taxing on my body too, but being the person that I am, I put my head down and kept pushing. I wanted to help others maneuver through Cancerville with support and resources. I could not stand the thought of another person choosing to die because they could not afford to live. But the reality was, and still is, the possibility of a reoccurrence is real for me too. Therefore, I found it difficult to live in peace when I had to face reoccurrences every day. After stepping away from serving clients, I found it manageable and understandable when I have random thoughts or dreams of a reoccurrence. Unfortunately, this will always be a part of me. There is no prayer or hymn, or anything else that will stop reminding me of this fact. So, what I have decided to do is live in every moment I get. Make the best out of every situation I find myself in. I don't live in fear, I push through it, although the thought of a reoccurrence does scare me. I live for Christ, knowing that what is to come can be dealt with, no matter what.

Now, after four years of being present for my family during Christian's critical developmental stages, we all agree it is time for me to share my story once more. In years past, I shared my story on many different stages through KSIBCF, personal request, and City of Hope. I had the opportunity to speak at cancer walks throughout southern California, donor events across the country, and a few of City of Hope's Spirit of Life Galas with up to 2,000 in attendance. Aside from meeting Florence Henderson a few years ago at a Spirit of Life Gala, the most memorable Gala was on October 11, 2018, honoring Mr. Jon Platt in the Music, Film and Entertainment Industry. This black-tie event was so star-studded it was like the Grammy's in October. Typically, I would have been escorted by Charles to an event of this caliber, but unfortunately, he was away on business in Texas. This opened the door for our miracle child, Christian, to be my escort. Although he did not like the formal attire, he was sharp as a tack.

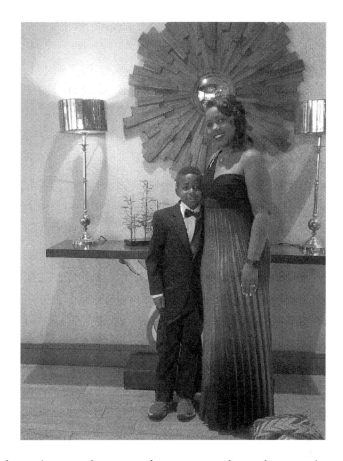

As the patient speaker, my role was not only to share my journey as a patient at City of Hope, but to make a personal connection with every person in the room. I needed them to know that their support changed lives beyond the patients they may see. I needed them to understand had I not known about City of Hope, I would not be standing before them. You see, the surgeon who performed the original biopsy was prepared to give me a lumpectomy the day he delivered the news. I can only assume that this was his way of trying to right a wrong as a result of his and my primary care physicians' error. As thoughtful as his gesture was, had I chosen to allow him to help me, I would have been signing my death certificate. As previously mentioned, Inflammatory Breast Cancer is a disease of the skin and the breast tissue. Had he only removed the tissue, unknowing, he would have left behind the cancer in the skin of the breast.

Sadly, I witnessed firsthand such a tragic mistake with two KSIBCF clients who did not survive six months after their lumpectomy. Not to mention the fact that my beautiful, healthy son was standing next to me on stage in a black tuxedo and Golden State Warrior blue kicks. He alone represented the generational impact every donor has contributed to. Statistically, the fact that I am still alive, 14 plus years later, is miraculous. But having a 10-year-old son with no ramifications from treatment, one could be rendered speechless, no matter who you are. My story, our story, is a story of impossible possibles that defied all the odds in so many ways and gives your heart and mind something ever so priceless, HOPE!

This particular night, I relived my journey through my words standing before an audience of 2,000 guests. I spoke from my heart and left everything on the stage, I allow myself to be vulnerable for the sake of HOPE!

According to Steve Baltin, a Contributor to Forbes.com, "Among the most powerful moments on this night was a moving speech from Kommah McDowell, a cancer survivor helped by City of Hope. She was as much a star on this night as music's unquestioned star of stars Beyoncé."

So, that same HOPE transcends my journey of the past and leaps into what is to come for mine and my family's future. It was at this event that I was encouraged by Jon and Angie Platt, Jermaine Dupri, Shawn and Beyoncé Carter, Usher, Kelly Rowland, Evan Lamberg, and so many more to go back to Cancerville and lend my voice, my passion, my expertise to the cause again. So, to them, I would like to say, *thank you*, for drawing me out of my bubble back into a world where there is so much that needs to be done.

As for my family, fortunately, our son is still healthy and strong. From birth, we knew there was something unique about Christian, our miracle child. Developmentally, he was very advance for his age as a baby and toddler. He walked, talked, and read books early. He is a very logical thinker, which is a blessing and a curse. Over the years he has tried several sports and for every sport he played, we were told he is an exceptional athlete. He learned to drive, drift, back up, and park a Power Wheel Corvette at the age of three; I have video to prove it, too. He began studying NASCAR races at the age of five and soon moved on to Formula 1 racing. He is an avid racing fan and he desires to be the first African American Formula 1 driver. As scary as this may sound to most parents, Charles and I are very supportive of Christian's career choice. He has had a burning desire to be a race car driver from birth. Only the Lord knows how far he will go, so in preparation, he has started his own racing company, C. McDowell Racing *fueled by Recycling*. Christian is the Chief Executive Officer; I serve as his Business Manager and Charles serves as his Financial Manager. For his 10th birthday, we bought him his first racing kart. Therefore, he is equipped to pursue his passion; however, he is responsible for fueling his passion, literally. Through C. McDowell Racing, he collects recyclables and cashes them in for fuel. This is an opportunity of a lifetime for our son and his hard work, week after week, proves he is fully vested in his dream.

Meeting in the Middle

"You will make mistakes, change your mind later on the wisdom of a decision, and hope to find better ways of doing something, but if you outline your values and determine the links to those values, the errors won't count."

Rose Marie Whiteside, As For Me And My House

Charles and I had been friends four years prior to him proposing to me. We talked freely about any and everything, including the type of person we thought we would marry, how many kids we wanted, and what we aspired to be as we crept up to the age of 30. We had no idea we were drawing the blueprints of our life together. Comically, we did not realize we were destined to marry each other until six months before the proposal. Our relationship was amazing because we shared our hopes and dreams without reservation. During pre-marital counseling, we took dozens of personality, compatibility, and character test, and we discovered that we were very similar in so many ways. Unlike many of our friends, the phrase *opposites attract* did not apply to us. However, we quickly learned even in our similarities, we went about things differently but ended up with the same result. This realization was pivotal to our relationship, as it would be tested over and over again. One of the most prevalent tests was our desire to have four kids.

Charles grew up in a close-knit large family with both parents, two siblings and cousins galore. I, on the other hand, was raised by a single mother, with one sister. Many of my cousins lived with us at one point or another, but most of my upbringing was just the three of us. So, with polar opposite family structures, we determined we wanted four children. Our rationale was, each one would have one to hang with. Of course, this was months before we would learn my fate. As time would tell, we were ever so blessed with

Christian. Unfortunately, I was not able to physically have any more children on my own, so we turned to adoption. Our desire was to continue building our family, if not through our blood, then through our love.... *different path, same result.*

Knowing that adoption is more than a notion, we proceeded with caution. We decided to go the route of Fos-Adopt. This allowed us to foster a child with the intention of adopting. After being approved as a Fos-Adopt family, we searched for a little brother for our son. We knew the process would take some time because we were very specific about the type of child we wanted to adopt. Interestingly enough, we found ourselves feeling uncomfortable with the process. Honestly, it felt like we were at a restaurant ordering food and we were a bit unnerved by this. But we learned through months of training, that our feelings were justified, and it was healthy to have realistic parameters for our child-to-be.

Unlike biological children, we were able to determine what we could or could not handle. We discovered that most children awaiting adoption had traumatic backgrounds, even at very young ages. Some children experienced trauma in the womb and the ramifications of that trauma was manifesting itself in their lives. We learned, many of the children were exposed to drugs of some sort and they bared the burdens of the side effects in their daily lives as well. We also learned having a sense of belonging is critical to having a stable mental space as kids develop. Many of the adoptable kids were not held at birth, thus causing a sense of disconnect in their minds. Other kids were abused physically or by neglect, which caused them to misunderstand healthy touch from someone who loved them or wanted to love them. Subsequently, trying to identify the type of child that would fit well with our family was challenging, nearly impossible. We did not want to be too specific, but we needed to ensure we could handle the traumatic weight that our son-to-be would be bearing.

Per Christian's request at 7 years old, we were looking for an African American boy with similar skin complexion to his. He also requested that his brother be one to two years younger than him. Charles and I, preferred an only child, however we knew that was unlikely. Knowing our son very well, we knew it would be best to include him and his thoughts in the process. We wanted him to know this was a family decision and his contribution mattered.

We were naïve to think our search criteria was broad, and the process would be quick. But, in actuality, the combination of our request caused us to have an even narrower search, which made it very difficult to find an available child. We learned early in the process that most children available for adoption had siblings. Also, trying to find a child within our age range did not make it any easier. So, we waited…

After two years of waiting, we finally attended an Adoption Fair, per the request of the adoption agency we were working with. We were so nervous to attend the fair because we did not know what to expect. The last thing we wanted was to walk into a room of kids needing a home and having to "pick one" like in many movies. Under those circumstances, we knew we would need a bus to take them all home. So, we prayed before heading to the Adoption Fair and when we arrived, we found that there were no children present at all.

After a brief presentation on what to expect from the Adoption Fair, we had the opportunity to speak with social workers from various counties in southern California. We were given the freedom to peruse through binders of available kids at our own pace. Several other families were in attendance as well, but it was nothing like the movies projected. We were relieved.

At first, we did not know where to start in the room, so we headed to the back of the room away from the other families. After given permission to pick a binder, we opened our first binder to find a picture of a beautiful little African American boy. His complexion was similar to Christian's, he had just turned five years old that day, he loved sports and going to church. His profile indicated that he had siblings, but he had been separated from them due to circumstances.

"We found him" we thought.

After two long years of searching, we finally found a little boy who met most of our criteria. We reviewed his profile further and we asked all the questions we could think of at the time. Not sure of the next steps, we made it very clear that we were interested in learning more about this little boy. The social worker assigned to that table was excited to see we were interested in one of his kids, but he wasn't sure if he was even adoptable. He explained that this particular child was in limbo and minutes before we approached the table, they just added him to the binders to see if anyone would be interested in him. So, the social worker wasn't sure of how to proceed at this point. He advised us to contact our adoption agency with the child profile information and the social worker would get back to the agency with the little boy's current status.

With this glimmer of hope, we visited each social worker's table and sifted through every binder, just in case we had more than one option. Sadly, he was the only one. That day we left the Adoption Fair excited about the possibility of finding our son-to-be. We eagerly waited for our adoption agency to update us on his status. Finally, a few days later, we were told he was adoptable. We were so elated!! We decided to not tell Christian about the possibility of a little brother just yet. We agreed to tell him once we figured out what the whole process entailed.

After what seemed like an eternity, we were ready to take the next steps in our fos-adopt process. But, to our surprise, we were told our Home Study was outdated, and we were out of compliance. This was devastating to us. We were very meticulous with our paperwork and we did everything we were supposed to do logistically to ensure our ducks were in a row when it was time. We had no idea items in our file had expired, had we known it would have been handled immediately. Consequently, we were very disappointed to learn that we needed to complete several trainings and update several certifications before we could be considered a family of interest for any child. We were livid with our adoption agency for not notifying us prior to this moment.

After nearly two months, we completed all necessary trainings and certifications and we were finally able to meet our possible son-to-be's social workers. It was at this disclosure meeting that we were supposed to be briefed on his full background so that we could make an informed decision. His social workers shared all that they were legally permitted to share, and we learned that he still had visitations and daily calls with his birth mom. This was concerning at first, but recent history dictated that visitations never happened, and phone calls were only one to two minutes a day. Not knowing if this was normal, we left the meeting ready to move forward. We were willing to accept the traumatic weight this young child was bearing, including limited birth parent contact. We were also advised that once he was in our care for three months, we would be able to officially file for adoption to stop all interactions with his birth family.

Understanding that we were utilizing a fos-adopt process, we would become his foster parents initially, then we would have to apply for adoption once he was under our care. In all the trainings we attend, this was an ideal process because it allowed adoptive families to bond with their child-to-be prior to adoption. Thus, making the Adoption Birthday very significant in their lives, which we agreed was very important as well.

As excited as we were, we knew we needed to pause, take a step back and really think things through. There was great discussion between Charles and

I, as well as my mother, who lived with us and was co-owner of our house.

Now, let me pause for a minute and provide a little contextual background regarding my mom, Shirley Mordon. This will allow you to understand the significance of her role in our family. In 2012, Charles and I asked my mom to come and live with us in Pomona, CA. The purpose of this arrangement, so we thought, was for all three of us to minimize expenses to become debt free. She, however, was motivated by something altogether different, me. I had recently finished radiation therapy and was on watch for a reoccurrence. By accepting our offer to live with us, she would be able to watch over me just in case something happened. My mom felt every ache and pain I felt. She watched me like a hawk and prayed for me continuously. After much consideration of our proposal, my mom rented her home in West Covina, CA and moved into our home in Pomona. For two years, we reduced our excess spending and we were intentional about every dollar made, saved, and spent. Finally, in 2014, we were debt free and proud of it.

With this freedom, Charles and I then decided we wanted a change of pace, so we sought out a new home in San Gabriel Valley. Unfortunately, we were not pleased with what we found in any of the surrounding cities, so we began looking further south. Then, in March of 2014, we found a new development in Oceanside, CA and we fell in love. After sharing our desire to move with my mom, she considered her options and decided to sell her house and join us in Oceanside. As we had hoped, within a few months we bought a brand-new house big enough for all of us to live comfortably, 10 miles from the beach. My mom, being a creature of habit, found this change challenging for the first three years. Unlike many in-law horror stories, we have heard, my mom stayed out of our business. She did not interfere with our relationship or how we parented Christian. She was an in-home nana, but she was not the default babysitter. She gave wisdom when asked, but if she strongly disagreed with a decision we made at any point, she would pull either one or both of us aside and lovingly let us know what she thought about it. She also has the gift of discernment, which we have found to be priceless over the years. My mom was an intricate part of our day-to-day lives. As a result, she was included in the decision to move to the next steps in the fos-adopt process.

Fortunately, we were all on the same page, so we proceeded. Charles and I were reassured that with consistency, structure and love, this particular child's outside forces would be manageable and he would eventually blend right in with a loving family. Thus, potentially extending our family to a family of four… which meant, *two down and two to go.*

A few weeks later, we had the opportunity to meet the little boy. We were so excited and nervous. We were not sure of what we were permitted to say or do. We didn't know if we should shake his hand or give him a hug. On the flip side, we didn't want to be disillusioned either. We needed to stay focused and not melt when we saw his big beautiful eyes. We needed to interact with him in a way that would help us to determine if he was a good fit for our family. Most importantly, we needed to know if he would jell well with Christian. Knowing Christian's personality, we knew our adopted son could not have a dominating personality, yet we wanted him to have a competitive spirit. It would be nice if he had a sense of humor, even if it was corny. Of course, we also had to consider his interaction with adults he was familiar with, like his social worker, and strangers, such as ourselves. Was he a flight risk or a willing victim? Was he respectful, did he listen to adults? All these things ran through our minds.

We arrived at the meeting spot early and waited for twenty minutes for the social worker and the child to arrive. Upon their arrival, we greeted them with a handshake and introduced ourselves to the little boy we saw in the binder. He was even cuter in person, I began to melt.

"Focus, focus..." I thought. "Was Charles melting too?" I hoped he was keeping it together better than me.

For an hour, we talked, played chase, laughed and melted even more. "He was perfect," we thought. Now, it was time for Christian to meet his soon to be little brother.

A week later, we surprised Christian with a trip to meet him. Unfortunately, mom had to wait a little longer because she was the nana and considered extended family, although she was in the home. After giving Christian the back story of what had already been done in the selection process, we told him that this was his opportunity to give his feedback. As we drove to the meeting spot, Christian asked several questions and eventually sat silent the rest of the ride. He was nervous, hopeful, and a little afraid.

When we arrived, we waited for ten minutes for the social worker and the little boy to arrive. When they arrived, we introduced Christian to his potential little brother, they shook hands. For an hour, the two boys played while we talked to the social worker. They hit it off very well and they physically looked like they could be brothers. Visually, he blended well with our family. We were so excited; our prayers had been answered.

After this visit we were encouraged to take some time to think about if we would like to move forward or not. We gave ourselves the weekend to pray, revisit his file, discussed the potential services needed, and most importantly, we tried to imagine how this little boy would add to our family. With that, first thing Monday morning, we confirmed our interest and were ready to move to the next stage in the process. The social workers were excited to hear they had a possible forever home for this little guy. To our surprise, things moved in lighting speed and two weeks later we were making room for a new member of the family. Understanding at this point, he was only our foster child, yet we were hopeful.

Harsh Reality

"We can't ever be sure what our kids will remember (or what we hope they'll forget), but I kind of think the everyday moments will be the most valued in the end."

Sarah Williams, Cupcakes On A Tuesday

Our son-to-be was with us for nine months. We quickly became consumed with his needs with frequent doctor appointments, dental appointments, counseling appointments, in home therapist several times a week, school meetings and interventions, and karate for both boys. Then, in addition to our insane schedule, we legally had to work in two-hour visits with his birth parent every two weeks. Due to location, this visit would take two hours to get to the meeting spot and two hours to get home. This was very exhausting for all. Charles and I were always fatigued, and Christian began fading into a shadow while our new foster son became our primary focus. Fortunately, my mom was very attentive. She kept a pulse on Christian and always found a way to let him know that she saw him and heard him when we were so distracted. She became his advocate and made sure we did not lose sight of Christian in the midst of planning things for our foster son. Mom jumped in to pick Christian up from school or a friend's house when we had to make six-hour visits on Fridays. Mom took him to school events when we were home making good on a punishment or at therapy meetings. My mom's role for Christian morphed into his lifeline with the family and Charles and I did not even notice. Mom was Christian's saving grace, but over time the distance became apparent. We realized things needed to change. Bound by our legal obligations in the fos-adopt process, we became very frustrated with all of the red tape. However, we were encouraged that all would change once our fostering status was switched to adoption status.

On two separate occasions, there were hearings set to transition us from fostering to adopting our son-to-be, but at the last minute they were both switched to status hearings. The first time we were livid. We didn't understand what caused the change and why the courts would not let us move forward. We were tired of the rat race we were in with all the "requirements" of the county that consumed our lives. We were tired of all the false promises our son-to-be was hearing from his birth parent and there was nothing we could do about it. We were tired, and it had only been three months.

Our son-to-be could be sweet as pie, but he was devilish at home, church, and school. On his first day of school with us, we received a phone call from the principal telling us our son had choked a little girl from behind for no apparent reason. We were so shocked by this news, we didn't know what to do or how to react. It was at this point that we realized we had our work cut out for us. Then, after the honeymoon stage, which was around the first transitional hearing, he really began showing his true self, or as I am told, "there was an awakening." We quickly learned that he had an uncontrollable temper and a yearning to belong. We informed all vested therapist and counselors, and for a few months, we focused on these two issues. Then, just when we thought we had a handle on things, he started physically attacking Christian. Every time we left the two of them alone in a room, he would literally jump on Christian and try to beat him up. Christian, being in karate, was able to defend himself so he didn't think anything of the initial attacks.

Finally, one day Charles and I walked in on the boys fighting. We separated them and began questioning them individually. We discovered that Christian was defending himself and our son-to-be was the aggressor. Christian went on to tell us that these attacks were happening every time we left the room, multiple times a day, and had been going on for weeks. We were taken aback by this news because we had no idea. Then, after questioning our son-to-be, he told us that he wanted to beat Christian up because Christian was bigger than him. He went on to tell us that he will be able to beat him up when he gets bigger and stronger. We were speechless and a bit in shock by this new information. So again, we informed his therapist and counselors so that we could address this issue.

After months of working through some of the traumatic events that had transpired within the first five years of his life, we were able to help our future son see the value of having a big brother. We implemented team building games and activities in our family time. We were intentional about pointing out how families work together and help each other and not hurt each other.

With his therapist, principal, teacher, and life coach's help, we used any and everything possible to demonstrate what a healthy family looked like and how healthy families treated each other. After a while, it was working. Our son-to-be's behavior began improving in school, church, and at home. We were excited to see the change for the better, but we knew we had a long way to go.

For four months we worked on various issues that surfaced with our future son. It was like playing tennis with emotions. We had to learn to know which ones to swat back and which ones to just let go. We discovered sometimes he lashed out because he did not know how to properly express himself. Other times, he was just being mean. We realized, it was our job to study our son-to-be and be able to determine what was intentional and what was unintentional. Ultimately, we needed to understand him the way we understood Christian. The drastic difference was, we raised Christian from birth and we understood his level of reasoning and his intentions. With our son-to-be, we had no idea what was triggering his thoughts or actions. We did not know if certain smells, words, type of people, dress, or anything triggered a traumatic memory in his little mind. We found ourselves constantly questioning his level of reasoning and his intentions.

Life was nothing like we thought it would be during the adoption process, which is often the case for adopting families. I recall a friend's advice prior to welcoming our foster son into our home. Being a former Social Worker and adopted herself, Ruth Gill, was very sincere.

"I know you want another son and I know you want to help a little boy get out of the system, but please promise me one thing… do not sacrifice your birth child, your miracle child, to save another child."

She looked me square in the eyes and went on to tell me how she had experienced parents forsaking their own trying to save others. She reminded me of how much of a blessing Christian was and that he is our miracle child, a gift from God. I never forgot her words and when things started taking a turn for the worse, I held tight to her sound wisdom.

In the sixth month of fostering, we had another hearing that was supposed to change our status from foster parents to adoptive parents. But again, one week before the hearing it was changed to a status hearing. This time we were not as upset. Instead, we had one eyebrow raised and figured God may have another plan for our future son and we were open to other possibilities.

So, after the hearing passed, another shocking incident occurred on the last day of school. One of the school aids was nine months pregnant and was due to have a baby within days. She had gone into the kindergarten class to say goodbye to the kids and to wish them well. The kids asked if they could touch her belly and she let them. They were so excited to hear she had a baby in her tummy and not a watermelon. Our son-to-be was in the mix of kids, giggling and laughing. Then, he was the last one to touch the aid's belly and with a straight face, he looked up at her.

"Can I kill your baby?" He said in a strange tone.

Unbelievably shocked, our son's instructional aide whisked him away from the other kids.

"What did you say?" She asked.

"I asked if I could kill her baby?" He repeated expressionless and then he smirked.

Fortunately, the pregnant aide could not understand him because of his undeveloped palette, so she did not know what he said and went on unaffected. His instructional aid, however, was mortified.

Shortly after, I received a phone call from the principal informing me of what happened. I was flabbergasted.

"How could he ask her that?" I thought. "I have to apologize..." I felt terrible and completely embarrassed.

Before heading to the school, I called Charles to tell him about the incident. We were both speechless. I then expressed how embarrassed I was to have to apologize to the aide for something so inexcusable. We were both saddened by this incident. I headed to the school to meet with our foster son's teacher. She explained what happened and how disturbed she was by his statement. I completely agreed, but as his mom, I needed to talk to him to hear his side of the story. Shortly after, we headed home after picking up Christian. I pulled our foster son aside and sat him down to talk about what happened. I listen patiently as he ran through the events of the day. He was proud of himself and wrapped everything up with, "it was a good day." At no point did he mention the incident, nor the aide for that matter. So, after he was finished with his report of the day, I asked him what he said to the aide with the baby in her tummy. Then, without hesitation and in a matter of fact way, he looked at me and cocked his head to the side.

"I asked her if I could kill her baby." He said.
My heart sank, but I kept my composure.

"Why would you say that?" I asked.

"Because I don't want her to have a baby." He said.

His little body stood tall and ridged as he was telling me his side of the story. He was looking directly into my eyes without even blinking. A chill ran down my spine. This was mind blowing to me and I too was disturbed. Again, we informed his therapist, counselor and life coach about this incident. Each one was shocked by his question and his reasoning behind it.

At this point, school was out for the summer and we were headed out of town for a 14-day family vacation that included a 7-day Disney Cruise. We thought this would be exactly what we needed to regroup as a family. Charles, my mom, the two boys, our nephew, and I, with 12 rolling bags, hopped a plane to Canada. The trip was both fun and exhausting. Both boys and our nephew had a wonderful time. There was so much excitement and activities 24/7, we refused to have any negative energy on this trip, so we increased our level of tolerance, which reduced the disciplinary issues we had to deal with. More importantly, we survived and we thought this would definitely be a game changer for us all. We bonded, explored, experienced new things together, talked, hung out, and played. We were building new memories together as a family, it was good, so we thought.

After returning from our vacation, we began noticing an increase in attacks from our foster son on Christian. Our foster son was even more aggressive, to the point of attacking Christian in front of us and my mom. It became so bad that we were not able to leave them in a room together without an attentive adult for any period of time. We were heart broken by this. This was not the plan.

We struggled with our reality and realized, there was so much more to this sweet boy than anyone could have anticipated. We began to doubt our decision to adopt, which was heartbreaking. We had invested everything into our son-to-be, time, resources, energy, and most importantly, love. We agreed things would be different if we did not already have a son, but under the circumstances, the words of my dear friend started to ring true.

"Do not sacrifice your birth child, your miracle child, to save another child."

Then, four days before our foster son's birthday, my mom took the boys swimming. While there, our foster son kept jumping on Christian's back while he was swimming. This was concerning because our little one was wearing a floaty, and Christian wasn't. So, for every time he would jump on him, Christian would be pushed down underwater. My mom told our foster son several times to stop because he could hurt Christian and possibly drown him. When I arrived, my mom was giving another warning to her foster grandson, with the threat of having to sit out of the pool while everyone else swam. After being briefed on his behavior, I called him to the edge of the pool. He paddled his way over in his floaty, he was so cute. I told him, "If you get in trouble one more time, you have to get out of the pool. No more warnings."

He looked me in the eyes to acknowledge me.

"Ok mom" he said before he swam off.

He swam toward the group of kids in the deep end of the pool where Christian was treading water. Then, before I could sit in my seat good, he had reached Christian and pushed him down by the shoulder. Christian was so caught off guard that he went underwater flaring his arms, trying to swim back up for air.

"We don't play like that, it's not funny." I yelled across the pool.

Not thinking there was a cause for concern for our youngest's actions, other than boys play, I sat comfortably in my chair. But, as soon as Christian resurfaced, his foster brother put his hand on top of his head and with all his might, pushed him back under the water. This time, he pushed him hard enough for Christian's feet to touch the bottom of the deep end. At this point, it became obvious that this was no game. Instinctively, I began running across the pool yelling for my foster son to stop and let him up. In a split second, so many thoughts ran through my mind... *do I jump in, should I keep running, will I make it in time*... Underwater, Christian began swinging his fist and fighting his foster brother off of him, while desperately trying to gasp for air. His head made it to the surface one more time and again, he was pushed back under the water flaring his arms and realizing he was fighting for his life.

By the third dunk, I had made it around the pool and snatched our foster son out of the water by his floaty. Christian came up for air and his friends helped him to the wall. I was so livid, I sat our foster son in a chair and had to walk away to calm down. The whole incident happened so fast, but it felt like slow motion. I was very unnerved by this, and again, Ruth's words flooded my head. I called Charles and told him what happened, he was so taken aback by it all. Now what were we supposed to do? We informed all the necessary therapist, counselors, social workers, and life coach.

We were at a crossroads in the fos-adopt process. When is enough, enough? With all the wraparound services he was receiving, nothing and no one stopped him for coming after Christian over and over again. Several of his care team members asked if he was aware of what he was doing? Maybe he was playing, they said. Maybe it was a misunderstanding. Sadly, after I calmed down and we had gone home, I asked our foster son, in front of his behavior coach, why he did what he did. He looked me in my eyes and cocked his head to the side.

"Because I wanted to hurt Christian." He said, emotionless and without hesitation.

Now this was the straw that broke the camel's back. We were not willing to sacrifice our birth child, our miracle child, to save another child. We wanted to build our family up, not tear it down. Enough was enough!

We discussed our decision to change courses throughout the night with my mom. In the morning, we notified the social workers. We explained the string of incidents that lead up to what we see as an attempted drowning and they were devastated to hear the news. They just knew that if anyone was going to be able to handle this sweet boy, it would be us. To their surprise, we couldn't either. Now, the question remained, where does he go from here?

Fortunately, it was discovered that a family member had been seeking him out over the nine months of being with us. This, we figured, was the divine cause for the changes in the court hearings. After a weeks' notice, a distant relative resurfaced and she was willing and able to bring him back into the fold of his own flesh and blood. This was very exciting news for us, yet disturbing at the same time. We were disturbed because, if we had moved forward with the adoption, we would have moved away from his biological family to allow us all an opportunity for a fresh start. He would have never known about this relative. One of our stipulations for fos-adopting was to only consider children who did not have a family to care for them. Not to snatch a child from his own relatives, who actually wanted him. So, ultimately, we realized, our choice to not move forward was a blessing in disguise. Our foster son is now with his healthy biological family, where he belongs.

For nine months, we were able to teach him so many things that he was able to take with him into his own family. He learned strategies to manage his temper, use his words when frustrated, say what he means and mean what he says, how to pray, memorize scriptures, identify three good things at the end of each day, ride a bike, tie his shoes, properly make a bed, thoroughly brush his teeth, swallow pills, not to cuss, and so much more. We loved on him more than he knew what to do with. Sadly, we tried to build our family, but things did not work out as planned.

Impossible Possibles

"It's always something, to know you've done the most you could. But, don't leave off hoping, or it's of no use doing anything. Hope, hope to the last!

Charles Dickens, Nicholas Nickleby

In reflecting on the past few months, I often wondered about how life unfolds. I think about people like Jay Z, Beyoncé, President Barak and Michelle Obama, Oprah, Ellen, Walt Disney, Thomas Edison, and The Beatles. All household names who have left a footprint on the lives of so many, but they were not all born into the lime-light. As children, they had no idea who or what they would become. They could not have even fathom how impactful, revered, or sought after they would be. Conversely, I think about people who win the lotto or multimillion-dollar jackpots. BAM!! In an instance, their lives change. Their influence change, their circle of friends change, their perspective on life changes.

In the midst of these thoughts, I also think about my journey and how it paralleled the aforementioned. Instantly, something happened that drastically altered my future forever. It wasn't glitz or glamour, it wasn't fame or fortune, No, it was cancer. Cancer stopped me dead in the tracks of my life. Cancer gave me a new perspective on life that caused me to think about my influences, and reevaluate my circle of friends. Cancer took center stage, while everything else was frozen in time. I was forever changed, regardless of how long my forever would be.

Although it was a great pleasure to meet and share heartfelt words with Jon and Angie Platt, Shawn and Beyoncé Carter, Jermaine Dupri, Usher, and so many more world renounced artist and producers, it was more exciting to share the dance floor with them. To see them as "normal" people sharing the love of a great song on the dance floor. Dancing shoulder to shoulder with Beyoncé, two stepping with Usher and next to Jay Z, and being given encouraging words from Jermaine Dupri to persevere and MAKE a difference. Not allowing "NO" to stop me on my journey. I realize, I may never cross paths with these icons again. But it was in that opportunity I found my inspiration to make a difference again. Entertainers, politicians, athletes, and some lotto winners alike, began their quest of hope as they chased their passion to make a difference in society in their own special way. They try to find their niche so that they can stand out in the crowd. They persevere, they win some and they lose some. But it is all par for the course. Me, I am fueled by the passion of self-advocacy, listening to one's instincts, gut, the Holy Spirit and always fighting for the underdog.

Ever since the first 5K I walked celebrating the completion of chemo treatments, I wanted to run a marathon. At the time, I had no idea how long a marathon was and naively, I thought the 5K was at least half of a full marathon. Prior to my first walk, I did not know any avid runners and everyone I encountered only talked about 5K walks and runs. So, in my mind, a marathon could be fairly easy if I were outside of treatment and had time to heal. Well, thankfully I kept this idea to myself and just made it number one on my bucket list of things to do. Years later, I learned the actual distance of a marathon, 26.1 miles. I could not believe it! There was no way I could walk, let alone run, 26.1 miles even if I wanted to. So, I erased completing a marathon off my bucket list. Then, after attending the City of Hope Spirit of Life Gala on October 11, 2018, I was reinvigorated and I personally challenged myself to do something that would seem impossible. I needed to prove to myself that I believed in myself and that with God ALL THINGS are possible. So, after being nudged by a friend, Jennifer Holleman, I signed up for a ½ marathon with only three months to train. I was terrified, but determined to simply survive and cross the finish line.

Day after day I trained, it was hard. Understanding, due to the high dosage of chemo I received in treatment 13 years prior, now it is difficult for me to stand for 25 to 30 minutes, let alone run. Also, with the lymph node dissections on both arms, I struggled with swelling and fluid buildup in my arms and back. My ankles stayed swollen, and my already irregular heartbeat pushed my heart to the limit. But, by hook or by crook, I was going to finish this race. Initially, I ran every day for eight weeks trying to make up for the months of training I was behind on. As a result, I blew both knees out and was forced to rest and ice them for two weeks. During this time, another friend, Christen Kemp, came along side of me and signed up for the half too. She, being a former athlete, found it a bit easier for her body to tap into its muscle memory. Whereas my body was trying to figure out what the heck I was doing and why. With her support and now two knee braces, we continued training three to four days a week. Some days my body felt amazing, while other days I struggled terribly. It was hard!

Then, nine days before the race, my knee went out on me again. I could not believe it! I was so frustrated. We tried doing a short run, but I couldn't even finish a mile, I was done. For seven days I rested and iced my knee and prayed that I would be able to just finish, even if I was the last person. Finally, on March 10, 2019, Christen and I drove to San Diego for our first half marathon. We were nervous and excited. I was scared that my knees would give out and I wouldn't finish, because that wasn't an option for me. I watched Christen and could see she was full of adrenaline and what we learned was "a runner's high". Me, on the other hand, I was afraid I wouldn't make it, then what?

After the national anthem they released runners in ten different zones. The faster runners were arranged to run ahead of the slower runners to minimize traffic jams with runners, joggers, and walkers. When it was our turn, our zone took off, and there we went. Christen was my rock during this race, our families came to support us at mile six and at the finish line. We finished the race in under three hours, I could not believe it! I cried tears of joy, this was another impossible possible for me. My mom was proud of me, my son was proud of me, but most of all, my Charles was proud of me. God knew we needed this moment. I DID IT! Now I was able to cross off my one and only bucket list goal.

So now what?

The Real Fight

I was never crippled until I lost hope. Believe me, the loss of hope is far worse than the loss of limbs.

Nick Vujicic

"When our men lose their hope of a future and purpose, you'll surely watch them die a slow death in front of you."

Nan Jones, The Perils of a Pastor's Wife

Over the years, I learned that once educated, donors were in full support of the mission of organizations like KSIBCF and BCS. With a growing client base as evidence and complete transparency, the last few years of KSIBCF were filled with birthing fundraisers that would sustain the organization to the end. Unfortunately, I had to dissolve KSIBCF and step off the stage of advocacy to focus on my young family. But the time has come for me and my family to represent life beyond treatment. My struggle today is as real as it was back in 2005, just with a new lens. The fact that I am still alive and well demonstrates the importance of surviving not only treatment, but the avalanche of bills that plummet you well after treatment. As well as the follow-up care that is required for the rest of your life.

I have found that the fight against cancer in many cases is surviving the treatment process. Many men and women are plagued with the debt of cancer, yet in this great country of ours, one would think there is more help for people during such a challenging time...

With all of the hundreds and thousands of walks, runs, marathons, and "a-thons" that take place from sea to shiny sea, you would think a patient and or family could get help through the treatment process without liquidating their life savings. Unfortunately, as a survivor, I learned that is not the case. Corporations tend to focus on research. Cancer research is the drive for the larger walks, runs, and *you name it*-a-thon. There is money to be raised from those directly and indirectly impacted by cancer and again, they seek out research as the means to make a difference in their community. However, corporations and large companies that host successful walks by pulling at the heart of those who want to support the *fight against cancer* don't realize that cancer research is supported by billions of dollars. Discoveries are being made, doctors are receiving great salaries, institutions are building great buildings, large national organizations are hiring more staff and acquiring more overhead in the name of cancer. But, with all due deference, who is helping the family, or more importantly, the patients in treatment?

When you look at all the money generated in the name of cancer, how much of it offers direct support to patients? So many patients miss appointments for treatment because they cannot afford to get to and from the clinic. Many patients choose to forego treatment because they can't afford co-payments. Thousands of patients have to rob Peter to pay Paul to survive the day-to-day challenges of living through treatment. Yet, the question remains, who helps the patient and family?

In 2005, I started KSIBCF on a mission to fill the gap in the Fight Against Cancer. From the moment we opened our doors to service clients, I quickly learned that the need was even greater than I could have ever imagined. Women choose not to have treatment because they realize how much it costs and do not want to leave their family with the debt of cancer. Mothers have to choose between feeding their kids or paying co-pays for treatment. Parents of children with cancer have to quit their jobs to be by their child's side while struggling to maintain a household during the process. It is unbelievable how much money is raised in the name of cancer. However, it is daunting how hundreds and thousands of families like these never see a dime of it during their battle. Small grassroot organizations funding patients in treatment are small fish in a big pond. The money they are able to raise isn't close to the national organization fundraising power. Sadly, the little money that is granted for direct client services just touches the tip of the iceberg.

So many corporations have restricted their funding to cancer research, which leads to tangible outcomes and a few great perks. Donors want their name associated with a drug that impacts cancer in a positive way or a procedure that proves to be successful. Donors love seeing their names on buildings as an added bonus for their donation. But what about saving one life at a time? What about helping to make sure a patient survives long enough to receive the miracle drug and doesn't stop the process because he or she can't afford it? How about sustaining a family, which could be their own employee, during the process so they don't have to liquidate their life savings to beat cancer? When I look at the Fight Against Cancer through this lens, it appears cancer is winning.

I could only imagine what the Fight would look like if 10¢ or even 5¢ of every dollar raised for research from walks, marathons, major fundraising events, and corporate sponsorship was donated to service organizations in the trenches with patients. This assistance would allow for the small fish to combat the challenges of treatment with families in the fight of their lives. I guarantee patient and family stress levels would drop, survival rates would increase, prognosis would improve, and personal outlook would also improve. Such funding would yield hope and give patients a fighting chance. The scales would be tipped in their favor and the belief of having children, watching their children grow old, seeing grandchildren, or witnessing a child getting married could become a reality.

When managing KSIBCF, I often sat at my desk and cried for those patients I had to turn away because the funds were exhausted. As they pleaded on the phone for help because they had no one else to help them, nowhere to go, and they can't believe they are going to be kicked out on to the streets all because they "got cancer". As sad as that may sound, the worst part of the call was when they said, "I have supported cancer walks for years and now that I need help, no one is able to help me!" Sadly, I heard this too many times and my heart broke every time.

Cancerville is real in so many ways and many patients and families reside there as they endure treatment. My hope is to shed light on the needs of the cancer world beyond research. To encourage donors to not only support research, but see the epidemic one person at a time. What good is research if patients give up before research can be brought to their aid? Sadly, there is no shortage of cancer patients, but those who are unable to afford the treatment process should not be collateral damage. Why wait for someone you love, or even you, to be in this position. *What if* we assisted with lodging for families in treatment? Lodging that would allow patients to be near their cancer treatment center? Lodging that would allow families to stay for free or at a minimal cost with their loved ones. *What if* we were able to assist with meals and transportation during their journey? Knowing it is the little things that matter most, *what if* we just did SOMETHING? Something to minimize the collateral damage. Imagine what we could do together?

Christian is ten-years old now and his mere existence represents life beyond treatment. To date, he has not demonstrated any side effects to my treatment. But Christian is here because Charles and I didn't give up and we had a support system that powered us through. There has to be a better way to give families in treatment a fighting chance to survive. We live the impossible, he is the impossible, and we know that anything is possible.

As a California State 76th Assembly District 2019 Woman of Impact, I charge those of you in the Fight Against Cancer to view the fight through a new lens. Cancer was the BEST worst thing that ever happened to me because it opened my eyes to what is truly possible, ANYTHING!

MAKE A DIFFERENCE

My family will support the Fight Against Cancer by donating $1.00 of every paperback book sold to organizations funding cancer patients in treatment.

Thank you for your support!

Kommah McDowell
aka Koko

www.KommahMcDowell.com

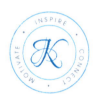

ABOUT THE AUTHOR

Kommah McDowell, MSLM, has a Bachelor of Arts in English, a Master of Science in Leadership and Management, and over 20 years of influencing change through motivational speaking. As a 14 year survivor of Triple Negative Inflammatory Breast Cancer, she is also an advocate for patients in treatment. She continues to serve the cancer community in various capacities.

75791658R00081

Made in the USA
Columbia, SC
24 September 2019